Sutras of the Inner Teacher

The Yoga of the Centre of Consciousness

Martin and Marian Jerry

Foreword by Swami Veda Bharati

Unlimited Publishing
Bloomington, Indiana

2M Communications
Canmore, Canada

Copyright © 2001 by Martin and Marian Jerry

Distributing Publisher:
Unlimited Publishing, LLC
Bloomington, Indiana
www.unlimitedpublishing.com

Distributed electronically by:
BookZone, Inc.
Scottsdale, Arizona
www.bookzone.com

Contributing Publisher:
2M Communications
Canmore, Alberta
Canada

Cover Design by Charles King
Copyright © 2001 by Unlimited Publishing, LLC

All rights reserved under Title 17, U.S. Code, International and Pan-American Copyright Conventions. No part of this work may be reproduced or transmitted in any form or by any means, electronic or mechanical, including photocopying, scanning, recording or duplication by any information storage or retrieval system without prior written permission from the author(s) and publisher(s), except for the inclusion of brief quotations with attribution in a review or report.

Excerpts from *Light on the Path* by Collins (1976) and the *Shri Yantra* are used by permission of the Theosophical University Press, Pasedena, CA. Excerpts from *The Yoga of Spiritual Devotion: A Modern Translation of the Narada Bhakti Sutras* by Prem Prakash (1998), Inner Traditions International, Rochester, VT are used by permission of the author. Excerpts from the writings of MaLa Sahan are also used by permission of the author. Figures courtesy of Rick Eden.

Unlimited Publishing, LLC ("UP") provides worldwide book design, production, marketing and distribution services for authors and small presses, serving as distributing publisher. BookZone provides worldwide electronic distribution. Neither BookZone nor UP exercises editorial control over books. Sole responsibility for the content of each work rests with the author(s) and/or contributing publisher(s). Information or opinions expressed herein may not be interpreted in any way as originating from nor endorsed by UP, BookZone nor any of their officers, employees, agents or assigns.

Previous edition published by 2M Communications, 2000.

Printed copies of this book are available at:
http://www.unlimitedpublishing.com/authors

Electronic copies of this book are available at:
http://www.bookzone.com/bookzone

ISBN 1-58832-029-4

Unlimited Publishing
Bloomington, Indiana

Dedicated to
Our Gurudev H.H. Sri Swami Rama,
And to our Spiritual Teacher Swami Veda Bharati

Contents

Preface — 11

Introduction — 15

I THE FOUNDATION — 33

The Centre of Consciousness — 33
1. Now begins instruction on how to work with the Centre of Consciousness. — 33
2. The Centre of Consciousness is the Inner Teacher, the Inner Guru. — 34
3. It is awakened through the grace of one's Spiritual Preceptor by initiation. — 35
4. The Spiritual Preceptor is a messenger whose task is to deliver the wisdom of the sages of the Himalayan Tradition. — 35
5. His or her task is also to introduce the qualified student to the teacher within. — 35

Adhikara: Qualification — 38
6. The Centre of Consciousness awakens only in the qualified student. — 38
7. Strict commitment to moral behaviour is assumed, both for qualification and even after the awakening of the Centre of Consciousness. — 41
8. Otherwise there is risk of a fall. — 41
9. The restraints (yamas) and observances (niyamas) of Raja Yoga form the core of morality. — 43
10. Ahimsa (non-injury), satya (truthfulness), asteya (non-stealing), brahmacharya (continence) and aparigraha (nonpossessiveness) are the yamas (restraints). — 44
11. Shaucha (purity), santosha (contentment), tapas (austerity - physical and mental discipline), svadhyaya (scriptural study and mantra repetition) and Ishvara pranidhana (devotion to God) are the niyamas (observances). — 47
12. Tapas, svadhyaya and Ishvara pranidhana when practised together constitute Kriya Yoga, which makes up the core of yoga at this stage of the Spiritual Path by providing the practice itself, the map to guide the journey, and the goal and guidance from the Centre of Consciousness. — 48
13. Ishvara Pranidhana, surrender to God, awakens with the Centre of Consciousness. — 50

The Personality — 51
14. The aspirant is body, breath, mind and soul or spirit. — 51
15. Manifested reality (the universe or the individual personality) is consciousness enrobed in energy arranged in layers within a vibrational spectrum ranging from matter through the subtle (pranic) body (which is accessed by breath), to several layers of mind. — 53
16. These interpenetrating energy fields of higher and higher vibrational frequency constitute the personality which is suffused with consciousness emanating from the core. — 53
17. The experience of physical matter is a construction of the five senses. — 55
18. Prana (subtle energy fields) is the missing link between mind and body. — 56
19. Breath is the gateway to control of the psychoneuroimmune system and host resistance. — 58
20. Svara yoga is the science of breath rhythms. — 60
21. All of the body is in the mind, but not all of the mind is in the body. — 62

22. *Mind continuously constructs your experience of reality through models of the world.* — 66
23. *Manifested reality is holographic. There is both a cosmic and an individual person. The microcosm reflects the macrocosm.* — 68
24. *The Centre of Consciousness from which consciousness flows in various degrees and grades lies at the core of the personality.* — 70
25. *The Atman or Self at the core is pure Consciousness. The ultimate reality is Consciousness or Spirit.* — 71
26. *The scientific study of spirituality is the scientific study of Consciousness.* — 72
27. *Yoga is the science of spirituality.* — 73

II THE EXPERIENCE — 76

Mystical Experience of the Centre of Consciousness — 76

28. *We are citizens of two worlds.* — 76
29. *The awakening of the Centre of Consciousness is a qualitatively new and unique experience in the inner world.* — 77
30. *It is possible to experience Spirit and not to recognize It.* — 78
31. *The initial experience of the Centre of Consciousness can be disturbing.* — 79
32. *The universe of manifestation is like one's own dream-creation, like an image reflected in a mirror.* — 80
33. *It is a secret that once revealed remains a secret.* — 81
34. *The Sages describe It as THAT. There is no substitute for direct Realization.* — 81
35. *The Centre of Consciousness is Consciousness-Without-an-Object.* — 82
36. *The Centre of Consciousness is a still, but effulgent, Conscious Presence, Silence or "Thatness". It is a Void or Emptiness that paradoxically is also a Plenum or Fullness. It pervades all of inner space and holds all manifestation, all inner mental content, within Itself like space pervades and holds the contents of a room, and yet is unaffected by them.* — 82
37. *Space is Self and Self is Space. In inner space the wise find the Intelligence of pure Consciousness, and ultimate Truth in the effulgent Void.* — 84
38. *From the Centre of Consciousness comes the gentle whispering of the Inner Teacher. Love whispers.* — 86

The Warrior Within — 88

39. *In consciousness the Inner and the Outer teachers are One and the Same.* — 88
40. *The Voice of the Master is the Voice of the Silence.* — 89
41. *The Inner Ashram has opened.* — 90
42. *Having been tested and found to be qualified, the student is accepted as a disciple. The Inner Teacher has responded with the grace of a Master.* — 90
43. *The relationship is eternal.* — 90
44. *The entry to the Path has at last been found.* — 91
45. *The Centre of Consciousness calls the student to discipleship.* — 91
46. *To cross over the threshold the student must die to the world.* — 92
47. *Total surrender and commitment are required, for the Inner Teacher ultimately is one's own Self.* — 92

III THE CURRICULUM — 93

The First Curriculum — 93
48. *Learn to walk in joy.* — 94
49. *Learn integrity in all things.* — 95
50. *Learn unconditional love.* — 97
51. *Learn the lesson of surrender.* — 99
52. *Learn that wherever you go, you carry the Light within.* — 101
53. *Learn to live with high inner energy flows.* — 102
54. *Learn the art of intuition. Herein lies the seed of Jnana Yoga.* — 104
55. *Intuition is the Voice of the Silence.* — 106
56. *One becomes a spiritual guide spontaneously.* — 108
57. *Learn to be selfish! Share what you have been given that you may receive more.* — 110
58. *Learn the art of conscious death.* — 113
59. *Learn the importance of positive thoughts and emotions.* — 115
60. *Learn the art of creativity and effective action.* — 118
61. *Accept that the disciple is protected by the Tradition. All is well; it really is!* — 120
62. *Learn discrimination in all things. Common sense is rather uncommon.* — 120
63. *Learn to accept responsibility for Who you really are. Claim your power.* — 120
64. *In learning to act from the Centre, use the power of "as if".* — 122
65. *Learn the art of unceasing worship. This is the essence of Bhakti Yoga.* — 124
66. *Learn never to take the Inner Teacher for granted. Learn to take the Inner Teacher for granted!* — 128
67. *Working with the Centre of Consciousness is practical.* — 129

IV THE ATTUNEMENT — 133

Attaining Spiritual Devotion — 133
68. *Attainment of the Centre of Consciousness is threefold.* — 133
69. *One is purification through detachment.* — 134
70. *One is unceasing worship with a still, one-pointed mind.* — 134
71. *Most important is the grace of God through the blessing of a great soul.* — 134
72. *Spiritual devotion is also Ishvara Pranidhana* — 136
73. *The experience of Ishvara is both personal and transpersonal.* — 137
74. *Enlightened Masters are manifestations of Ishvara.* — 138
75. *Hiranyagarbha alone is the teacher of yoga.* — 138

Transpersonal Visioning: The Art of Loving Wisdom in Action — 139
76. *Understand the creative power of paradigms.* — 140
77. *To radically change your life the most powerful thing you can do is to change your models of reality.* — 140
78. *Generate a life vision of extraordinary beingness under the guidance of the Centre of Consciousness.* — 142
79. *Perform actions established in yoga.* — 143
80. *You can only create what you can imagine.* — 145

81. Recreate yourself under the guidance of Spirit in increments until your life vision of extraordinary beingness is fully manifested.	147
82. Transform your identity.	147
83. Recreate your life context.	150
84. Alter your way of evaluating what is real.	153
85. The universe restructures itself to fit your new models of reality.	156
86. Follow your Centre without wavering.	157
87. Karma Yoga is action flowing from the Centre of Consciousness.	158

Meditation 161

88. With the opening of the Centre of Consciousness meditation moves from method to experience, from doing to being, from effort to absorption.	161
89. With the opening of the Centre of Consciousness meditation moves from activity to communion, to at-one-ment.	163
90. The three-fold distinctions of subject-object consciousness collapse into the unity of absorption.	165
91. Meditation gradually becomes spontaneous.	167
92. There are yogas of life and yogas of discipline.	167
93. Meditation is the beginning and the end of all of these.	168
94. There are as many Paths as there are Pilgrims.	171
95. The mantram comes from and goes back to the Centre of Consciousness.	173
96. In the Centre of Consciousness, love, wisdom and action are unified.	174
97. From the Centre of Consciousness flow both witnessing awareness and awareness with intent.	174
98. Surrender all practice to the Centre of Consciousness.	176
99. Life becomes a living meditation.	176

V THE BLESSING 180

The Opportunity 180

100. To come under the guidance of a Master is a blessing rare, and of the Inner Teacher, rarer still.	180
101. Learn to take the essence of such a life	181

The Essential Path 182

102. The core practices for the Path are now five:	182
103. Act with unyielding integrity and discrimination through moral behaviour as guided by Spirit, as though death were looking over your shoulder.	182
104. Develop quietness, calmness, stillness, tranquillity and equanimity of mind, breath and body.	182
105. Purify the personality through worldly detachment and surrender to the Centre.	182
106. Develop a one-pointed mind.	182
107. In all conditions and through all experiences meditate with unceasing worship of the Centre of Consciousness.	183
108. But foremost is the grace of the Master, the Inner Teacher.	183

End Notes 185
1. *The neurophysiology of emotions* 185
2. *Psychoneuroimmunology* 190
3. *Neurocardiology* 191
4. *The holographic universe* 193
5. *The scientific study of consciousness* 195
6. *Consciousness in Advaita Vedanta* 208
7. *Subpersonalities* 209
8. *Death* 211
9. *Life Planning* 216
10. *Background Visioning* 221

Glossary 225

Bibliography 231

Index 239

Preface

Sir Isaac Newton perhaps read, or came across a reference to, the ancient Indian *Vaisheshika* philosophy which stated in the 4th century B.C. that the falling of a fruit (no apple was mentioned) downwards is the proof of the force called *gurutva* (Prashasta-pada's Commentary on the *sutra*s of Kanada – i.e. *one who ate atoms for grains*). Thereafter 'gravity' (an abstract noun, derived from Sanskrit *gurutva*) was no longer confined to a situation but, as a proper noun, began to denote a particular force.

It is thus that words change their meanings – the same old words expressing newly discovered truths. This is even more so with spiritual discoveries. However, nothing new can ever be discovered about the realities spiritual. What is perennial resides in every soul, and has been stated many times over by the sages, the realised ones. One to whom the perennial has become real is a realised one because thereby s/he has become real to oneself, shedding the theretofore falsehood of the notions about the self.

Realisation or enlightenment, replacing darkness and stupor with light and an awakening, is not a sudden one time event. It is a gradual unfolding, unveiling, raising the volume of light. It happens by degrees. Each day in the life of a spiritual seeker is a day of enlightenment, compared to the previous day. Each tree under which he sits to rest during his journey is a *bodhi* tree.

Many changes occur in such a pilgrim from time to time. One of these is that s/he uses the same old conventional words in a more and more refined sense to express an elevated state.

Similarly the changes occur in the conventional usage of words in the society. Some words deteriorate in meaning, like the words *holocaust* and *apocalypse,* as certain elements in the society darken. Some words gain in glory, for example "to sit" in the meditative circles no longer means just sitting down for any purpose, but to meditate. "To breathe" is no longer merely a biological involuntary function but refers to meditating with breath awareness. Independence does not mean 'of the republic'; freedom does not mean 'from slavery', liberation is not of a certain social class from the bondage of another class These are words imbued with the content of the highest spiritual goal, a freedom not 'from' or 'to' a condition but *moksha*, spiritual liberation that is not dependent on a condition that is its antecedent or its consequence. It **is**. By itself, within itself, *sui ipse, sui generis, svayam-bhu.* Upon being in that, one is no longer in bondage of another nation, class, personage, or condition externally imposed.

A Sanskrit text on mathematics may use the word *bindu* in the sense of its cognate *the point*. But someone dwelling in the one-pointed mind is centred in that point of ineffable light for which every awakened one serving humanity remains intensely nostalgic. So also the word *centre*. In the spiritual realm it is not a centre of something other than itself. It *is*. That is the *point*, not *of*, but that *is* the *centre of consciousness*. The centre of consciousness does not evolve, does not shift, does not appear or dis-appear, submerge or emerge. It is has no relevance to particles like 'if', adverbs like 'where' and 'when'. One does not say 'when I was liberated'... "It is qualitatively new and unique" only from the point of view of those who are not yet *within* it.

As the spiritual height unveils itself, its experience seeks compassionately to spill over for the benefit of others who are yet in the valley. This spillage has to take the form of words. It picks out the words already in vogue and changes their usage and meaning. There is an immense body of literature in Sanskrit discussing these language-formation processes. The reader of the *sutra*s published here will find that the words familiar to him have a meaning other than the ones in common usage. The psychologist will see herein states of the shallow layers of the mind sea that s/he has delved in. A therapist will look for application to disturbance and disease. The philosopher will speculate in his terminology. The Socratic and the Platonic will see one truth, the Kantian some other. But, as the poet Tagore says :

> From the word of the poet men take what meanings please them,
> but their last meaning points to *Thee*.

The last meaning of these *sutra*s is simply the Nature of Divinity within us. It is no mere speculation presented as a hypothesis. The Master always spoke of seeking personal experience. What is stated here is experiential. Even a distant glimpse of this light fills the soul and then spills over, as it has done herein.

Drs. Martin and Marian Jerry tell me that they went to see the Master for the first time, with a long list of questions. Each time they would open their mouths to ask a question, they would be interrupted by the Mater saying " I will answer *aaalll* your questions". This went on for several days until it was for them time to leave the Presence. They were not able to express any of their questions, and came back somewhat puzzled. The questions are never answered; they are resolved – and that is the answer within. Thus does the Guru within answer them. The answers thus received are recorded herein.

I pray that you read these not according to the conventions of your usage of the language but what the words are actually meant to convey of the experience.

May the gravity pull (*gurutva*) of the Teaching Spirit (*guru-tattva*) draw you and guide you to the same first hand experience.

May the presenters of these answers here one day reach the status of a *rishi*, the ultimate in the accomplishment of intuition in yoga.

Swami Veda Bharati

Swami Rama's Ashram, Rishikesh, Dec.30, 1999.

Introduction

Samahita Yoga: The Yoga of the Centre of Consciousness

We have powerful memories of our first meeting with our spiritual preceptor, H.H. Sri Swami Rama of the Himalayas. Our spiritual teacher, Swami Veda Bharati, insisted on such a meeting, and at the time we were puzzled as to why it was necessary. But it soon became apparent that a meeting should take place, so we wrote a letter to request one. Immediately a reply came from Swamiji (as he was affectionately known by all his students and disciples), through his secretary that he would meet with us. We had a long distance to travel across the North American continent so that two days would be required just for the travel. We arranged for a short retreat at his ashram over a weekend, and we were astonished at how the whole world seemed to stop to allow us to go. We were both very busy health-care professionals and solidly in the middle in the sandwich generation with responsibilities for two children as well as aging parents. This weekend turned out to be the only weekend that entire summer that our responsibilities were taken care of so that we could both be free to go. The journey began auspiciously when we were bumped to first-class on the flight. After arriving at the ashram we requested the appointment with Swamiji and were given a time and place to wait.

Swamiji came down the hall to meet us, a huge man in dark robes who towered over us. Taking our hands, he held our eyes with his and said three times, "I will answer all your questions." Little did we know until very much later that this was our first introduction to the Inner Teacher and to the ultimate promise of *samadhi*. For Swamiji defined *samadhi* as the state in which all questions are answered and no questions remain.

> "The word *samadhi* means *samahitam* - no question remains unanswered, no mystery remains unsolved."
> Swami Rama, 1999a

We choose to coin the term, *samahita yoga,* to describe the Yoga of the Centre of Consciousness, which is the focus of this book. It honours the profound impact of our first personal experience of our Guru, and what was to become the essence of our teaching from him in this lifetime.

The nature of the Centre of Consciousness and how to work with It will be explored in detail in the sutras. Briefly, we are referring to the Inner Teacher, the inner guru, the teaching spirit in the universe or *Hiranyagarbha* in the yoga tradition. Parallel concepts would include the Holy Ghost or Holy Spirit of the Christian tradition, or the *Sambhogakaya* in Buddhism (Arya, 1979a). We use the same term that Swami Rama so often used - Centre of Consciousness.

One teaches what one needs to learn. The exercise of writing of this book was as much for our benefit as for you, the reader. In that sense it is a purely selfish exercise, for if one wishes to have spiritual knowledge then one is obliged to give it away. The underlying belief or assumption behind this statement is key: it must be a part of your essential being or you could not have it to give away. All of this sounds very New Age. But Karma Yoga is actually the yoga of manifestation to use more modern language. That is why we act - to bring will, intent and desire into manifestation.

The Promise of the Millennium

For the last two to three decades much has been written about the new millennium beginning in 2000 AD. (Although actually the new millennium begins on January 1, 2001). Many of these prophecies are very old. Most of them are foreboding. As part of the New Age the more recent writings describe various versions of some kind of planetary transition involving everything from shift of the earth's poles through to alteration of its magnetic grids. The effects of these major events have been forecast with various degrees of cataclysm as the earth adjusts, such as earthquakes, severe weather and volcanic activity with their attendant devastation to the population at geographic risk. We have certainly seen such events during the close of the decade of the 1990's, but there is real argument as to whether their severity is any more or less than previously in history. Swami Rama said little about this, other than that such major transitions have occurred on the planet many times in history.

In addition to a physical planetary transition of some kind to take us into the New Age and the new millennium, the prophecies also predict an age of greater spirituality. The term "ascension" is often used in the writings to describe the awakening of spirit within humankind and the attendant radical transformation and raised vibratory rate of the personality. This word "ascension" is used in various ways. Some writers envisage a scenario like the Christian rapture with waves of individuals going through this radical spiritual transformation during the early years of the new millennium (e.g. Redfield, 1993; Carroll, 1998). Because of the earth changes, particularly of the magnetic grids, coupled with the subtle energetic pathways cut by the saints and sages of yore as they reached enlightenment in the past, some say that it will now be easier than ever in the earth's history to achieve full spiritual realization. The bonds of karma will be more easily shed. Indeed some are of the opinion that the high earth population, recently having reached six billion, is representative of the presence of many beings who wish to avail themselves of this unique opportunity for spiritual advancement.

Still others use in the word "ascension" to indicate the acquisition of self-realization at the point of death when the soul is freed of the restrictions of a physical vehicle. Also, some use the term "ascension" to represent what has traditionally been called yoga and self-realization or enlightenment in the perennial wisdom (MSI, 1996).

Then there is a more traditional viewpoint that recognizes how little people change in a single lifetime, even with a modicum of practice with a spiritual discipline. This more traditional view sees the spiritual path as extending over numerous lifetimes. The process might remind one of the exponential growth of money with compound interest. With each calculation of interest one takes into account both principal and the interest accrued to that point. The curve of accumulation of money starts to rise very slowly over quite a long period initially. In the final stages the curve begins to rise very steeply, building on the solid base of accumulated investment that the exponential process provides.

The spiritual path is analogous. In the perennial wisdom a curve representing accumulating spiritual progress would extend over many lifetimes. The gain of each lifetime forms the foundation for the accomplishment in the next, the individual beginning where he or she left off in the previous lifetime. When one works with a spiritual master or guru, that meeting may take place after one has paid off the major portion of that particular lifetime's karma. Then one is relatively free to take up the study of the path with the master where one left off to go on to the next step in progress for that lifetime. As one progresses along the curve it rises more and more steeply, representing more being accomplished more quickly with each lifetime, beginning earlier and earlier. Once that solid foundation is in place then the process becomes very rapid in the matter of a lifetime or very few lifetimes to completion.

It is often asked whether one can be enlightened in a single lifetime. The answer is yes, but it assumes not only a single-minded application to spiritual practice and the good karmic context to make that possible, but also the existence of that long foundation of preparation from prior lifetimes. If one uses the term "ascension" in this respect, then it is consistent with the more traditional model of the perennial wisdom and yoga as the science of spirituality.

Our point in bringing this up, quite simply, is that the science of yoga is the original "ascension technology". Over the centuries and millennia it has produced a long line of enlightened saints and sages in various traditions of its expression. It has a track record of success. Whether the scenarios of planetary shift and ascension into New Age occur or not, the practice of yoga as the science of spirituality is the best assurance of success on the spiritual path if this is what the student wants. The student of true yoga (and not some of the artificial variants that pass as yoga in the West), can be assured of a valid method with a long history of demonstrated success. He or she will be prepared for whatever may or may not occur as a planetary shift or a New Age of spiritual transformation.

Many of the techniques for ascension being offered in the New Age writings currently may or may not be efficacious for they are untried and lack the pedigree of success that yoga has. If you want ascension technology, however you may define the word "ascension", look to authentic yogic teachings as the best foundation. Once the Centre of Consciousness opens you will have individual guidance as to how to build on that foundation.

We dearly wish that we could give you the experience of the Centre of Consciousness. But we cannot. The opening of the Centre is a matter of divine grace. The purpose of this book is to provide some practical guidance on how to work with the Centre of Consciousness once it opens. If the prophecies of spiritual awakening are true then many will need help on how to cope with this opening. Perhaps this book will be timely and prove helpful at least to some who may wonder what is happening inside themselves.

This process of awakening is natural. Indeed, some would say that it is human kind's next major evolutionary step for the species (Gopi Krishna, 1971). But because it introduces qualitatively unique and unprecedented inner experiences, it can present problems to those who are unaware of what is happening to them.

One individual, for example, experienced great anxiety and panic attacks, thinking he was losing his mind. Another felt paranoid with the sense that something was watching. A young woman had a deep experience of awakening which was transient. She then felt that God had abandoned her and suffered severe depression for ten years. Another individual who had a profound experience of that awakening decided he was enlightened, was convinced he could induce the same state in others because he had it, and began to advise others that there was no further need for spiritual practice or meditation.

This experience should not be confused with enlightenment or with the experience of raising the kundalini. It means only that the Inner Teacher has opened, that the years of long preparation have been successful, and that finally you have found the entry to the true spiritual path. There is a growing literature about transcendent experiences and how they are often confused with psychosis (Nelson, 1994; Grof and Grof, 1989, 1990). Some of this material is very helpful, but unfortunately much of it is confused regarding the nature of spiritual experience.

If the millennial prophecies turn out to be nonsense, the serious aspirant will still succeed on the path of an authentic tradition of yoga. If, on the other hand, the millennial prophecies turn out to be true, authentic yoga is still the basic science of spirituality and technology for ascension to cope with the New Age.

Why a Sutra Format?

Quite simply, this is the format in which the text was given to the authors. In meditative communion with the Centre the material simply flowed as fast as it could be written down. In New Age jargon this might be called channelling the Centre of Consciousness. In the yogic paradigm it is the intuitive revelation that characterizes communion with the Centre. We have great respect for material given in this way - that it be presented as purely as possible. We function simply as messengers, not as teachers who "know". The material is necessarily both coloured and enriched by its transmission through our own personalities and cognitive structures, especially in some of the commentary. The perennial wisdom is a unity; this is merely a particular expression of a portion of it that will be helpful to some at a particular stage on the Path.

Because of the role of intuition, read the book between the lines, from the heart. Rather than gulping it down, sip it a little at a time, digesting each bit thoroughly as you go. But be prepared now and then at some places in the commentary to switch gears from heart to head as we bridge East and West by adding some current science. Bridging East and West this way was part of our Guru's mission. To ease these transitions we have placed longer scientific commentaries as end notes identified by numbers, such as (1).

The sutra format is unusual in western writing. But in this context it becomes quite practical. The material presented is very difficult to summarize in a logical, linear fashion, the way western texts are usually written. Each sutra becomes a potent condensation of the essence of an essential point of the teaching. A sutra is a pointer to an internal intuitive mental gestalt that represents that teaching. The sutra awakens that gestalt within you, the reader, triggering its intuitive revelation into the mind from the Centre of Consciousness. For that Centre is available to us all whether we are aware of it yet or not. Contemplation is a process for unlocking the layers and layers of meaning lying potential within a sutra.

While the book can be read from cover to cover, you will extract most from it if it is used as a stimulus to contemplation. As you dip into its richness over and over it will provide increasing stimulation to the awakening of your own intuitions as whisperings from the Centre of Consciousness. It is in this sense that we want the book to be useful. The sutra format is very practical for this kind of material. It aids study, it summarizes, and it awakens contemplation.

Intuition and Revelation

Intuition means many things to different people. It is often confused with biological instinct or with emotions and feelings, or even with impulsive behaviour. In the West it is ridiculed as irrational and unscientific. It lacks respect as a reliable way to "know". We worship rationality and the intellect instead. But this text has intuition as its major focus.

In the realm of spirituality intuition is the primary way to know Truth, using the mind like a sixth sense. All of us have access to the intuitional faculty to varying degrees. But here we are talking about a direct conscious access to the wisdom that flows by revelation from the Centre of Consciousness, from Spirit. At a certain stage of spiritual path one simply cannot progress further without that inner guidance. With time intuition becomes the primary way to know Reality and Truth.

The Tradition of the Himalayan Masters

This text is based in the yoga of the Tradition of the Himalayan Masters, of which the late H. H. Sri Swami Rama was the most recent master to embody the full spiritual tradition in service to the external world. The home of the great spiritual traditions has been the Himalayan Mountains for millennia. Protected by the vastness of these awesome peaks the great sages have lived and passed on the knowledge of the teachings of yoga to generations of disciples who, in turn, have themselves become masters passing on the teachings in an unbroken master-disciple lineage since the Vedic period. In yoga it is common to ask a student to what tradition he or she may belong and its pedigree or lineage. The

Himalayan Tradition is an oral one of master-disciple transmission that can be traced back through records of generations of guru-disciple relationships for over 5000 years.

Ultimately there is only a single spiritual tradition (Tigunait, 1993). But like the trunk of a great tree giving rise to many branches, many manifestations of spirit have been expressed on this planet over the centuries. The Himalayan Tradition is considered to be one of the root or primary expressions of spiritual knowledge (Swami Veda Bharati, 1998). The lineage includes the great sage Shankaracharya who formulated the basis of Vedanta 1200 years ago. He organized his teaching into five centres within the Himalayan Tradition. Our particular tradition is the Bharati lineage as one of those five. The word "Bharati" describes one who is a lover of knowledge and who becomes totally absorbed in its light.

The teachings come not from a self-proclaimed teacher but are contained in the writings of the Tradition and the records of the experiences of its great masters. These teachings support a student's learning and help to explain the offerings of its teachers. The teachings are an independent body of knowledge to which the student can refer for explanation and confirmation of his or her progress, rather than just the personal authority of a single teacher. In this sense yoga is a spiritual science and it is taught as a science. The student is given the methods and the philosophy and then invited to prove their truth by self effort.

The purpose of the Tradition is to awaken the divine flame within each human being. The Inner Teacher is the first expression of the piece of divinity that all human beings carry within them. It is to the awakening of this Inner Teacher that this text is directed. Ultimately the goal for each student is to know his or her true self, to be able to answer from experience the question, "Who am I?" In this way eventually each student will become a master in the Tradition and will pass on the lineage in turn.

The role of a master in the Himalayan Tradition is to introduce the student to the Centre of Consciousness, the Teacher within. In performing this task of transmitting the lineage, the grace of the guru is expressed in initiation. This is an initiatory tradition. Indeed in the Tradition a guru is defined as someone who can give higher initiation (*shaktipat*). The passing on of spiritual knowledge is done experientially through higher and higher grades of initiation involving the transmission of spiritual energy. This whole process is called *transmission* and is the central focus of the Himalayan Tradition.

The Himalayan Tradition is based in Patanjali's *Yogasutras* or Raja Yoga as expanded by the methods and philosophy of the Tantras and Vedanta. These are combined with specific oral instructions and initiations that have been passed on by a long line of saints and masters of yoga. This is not an intellectual attempt to combine separate systems. Rather it is a unified and integral yoga that incorporates both the yogas of life and the yogas of discipline into a unified system of practice.

Our text is addressed to advanced students of the Himalayan Tradition to provide assistance at a certain critical stage of the unfolding of spiritual Consciousness on the Path. It assumes a basic knowledge of yoga as taught in the Himalayan Tradition and some practical familiarity with its practices and methods. But there will be something of value for every reader interested in yoga and spirituality

The first part of the sutras will review key aspects of this foundational knowledge in the context of the awakening of the Inner Teacher. It will provide the student with useful maps of inner space to guide the unfolding experience.

The Chariot of Sadhana

What then is *samahita* yoga, the Yoga of the Centre of Consciousness? In the first *pada* of Patanjali's *Yogasutras* considerable emphasis is given to two concepts that lie at the core of the practice of yoga at that stage of the Path. The first is *abhyasa* or practice, and the other is *vairagya* or detachment.

Swami Rama often spoke of the chariot of *sadhana*. One wheel is *abhyasa* and the other is *vairagya*. Both must revolve simultaneously for the chariot to progress. These two concepts are integrated into a third called *Ishvara pranidhana*, which is also given much attention in *pada I* of the Yogasutras. In what we call *samahita* yoga all three concepts are integrated into practice flowing from the experience of the opening of the Centre of Consciousness. Rather than something entirely new, this is simply an altered emphasis of Himalayan yoga particular to this stage of the spiritual path. Like the Himalayan Tradition, *samahita* yoga is anchored in the eight-limbed Raja Yoga of Patanjali. It also uses meditation as the core technique. But the practices must be reinterpreted with the opening of the Centre of Consciousness, which gives them an altogether new meaning and experience. The yogas of life are also integrated and we will show how they become unified in the Centre and in everyday life.

Abhyasa and Attunement With the Centre of Consciousness

In *samahita* yoga *abhyasa* carries the connotation of attunement with the Centre of Consciousness. Meditation begins to encompass *Ishvara pranidhana* or practicing the presence of God (in this case, practicing the presence of the Presence), including meditation in action. *Abhyasa* integrates all three yogas of life into practical daily living. Bhakti yoga provides the internal arc into the Centre while Jnana Yoga underlies its output as the wisdom of intuition into the mind. Karma yoga becomes action flowing from the Centre of Consciousness. The Inner Teacher becomes the loving centre or focus of all action and knowing.

Vairagya and the Technology of Detachment and Surrender

Swami Rama was a highly skilled adept, yogi and sage who was trained in the cave monasteries of the Himalayas, and to whom later was passed the full spiritual power, authority and knowledge of the lineage of the Himalayan Masters. In the 1970's his own master gave him the mission of bridging East and West, spirituality and science (Tigunait, 1998). Swamiji was told to teach the universal message of the sages to the whole world in a way that would bridge East and West. He was to teach only what he had personally practised and to see whether science was able to verify it. Swamiji was to create a second bridge - between science and spirituality, for both seek the source of happiness, one in the external world and the other internally. Through technology science provides for the physical needs of humankind, while spirituality nurtures the mind and the soul. When they become isolated as two solitudes, spirituality contracts to religious dogma and science becomes uncaring and materialistic.

This bridging of East and West became a key aspect of his global mission. We also believe that there is an urgent need for this East-West synthesis. Our own professional training in research and clinical practice in the medical and psychological sciences is reflected in the commentary on some of the sutras where we summarize parallel concepts in western science. Where appropriate, some of these concepts are developed in more detail in the end notes.

A key aspect of yoga and of the Himalayan Tradition in particular, is emotional and mental purification. Here western science can now provide considerable information on the physiological and biochemical effects of yoga practices such as meditation and pranayama. New concepts such as psychoneuroimmunology, the role of the brain in the heart (neurocardiology), and the psychosomatic network provide useful models. Therapeutic yoga is coming of age.

We also make reference to the role of visual-kinesthetic dissociation as key to understanding how practices like *antar mouna* and meditation purify the emotions and the mind.

Serious meditative practice can bring up much negative material in the process of mental and emotional purification. Recent advances in energy psychology - the so-called meridian therapies - can rapidly resolve such material without pain. Purification in yoga need not entail severe suffering any longer.

Often yoga is portrayed as a process of purification alone. Once the mind is purified of emotional and mental noise and can be stabilized in one-pointedness and stillness, then the effulgence of the Self will manifest spontaneously. This conceptualization is an "away from" strategy - a moving away from what is not wanted; a kind of backing into the spiritual centre. In fact this strategy does not work as usually conceptualized. The universe tends to give you, metaphorically speaking, what you pay attention to. Pay attention to suffering and you may get more of it.

With the opening of the Centre a new and increasingly dominant influence comes into play. Now the aspirant turns toward the Centre and moves "toward" what he or she wants and seeks as the primary process. The purification continues, but more as a surrender, with a natural falling away, atrophy or release of impurities.

To understand the change in mental and emotional content we discuss in depth the concept of models of the world or cognitive paradigms. These describe the mental structures by which the intellect makes meaning of experience and creates a personal experience of reality. A familiarity with this process from modern psychology, such as Neuro-Linguistic Programming and similar disciplines, becomes essential to understand mental paradigms and how they shift, the values and belief systems with which Consciousness identifies to create the small self and which form its bondage.

Surrender and relaxation are fundamental at all levels of the personality in Himalayan yoga where they are expressed in the posture of *shavasana* as a series of intricate methods for relaxation and for *yoga nidra* (yogic sleep). Thus release at the physical and energetic levels of the personality occur with methods like progressive relaxation or *yoga nidra*, which can be enhanced with the use of applied kinesiology and energy psychology. And release at the mental level occurs through meditation and related exercises, largely in relationship to their effect in producing visual-kinesthetic dissociation.

All of this is what we mean when we speak of *vairagya* in relation to the technology of detachment and surrender. It is perhaps in this one area that western science can provide much assistance.

Meditation: The Core Technology

Meditation is central to the Himalayan Tradition. Indeed it is said that all methods of meditation ultimately can be traced back to the Himalayan Tradition. In *samahita* yoga meditation plays two central roles. The first is attunement to the Centre of Consciousness, both to move into the Centre and to receive the intuitive and other outputs from It. This is the role of meditation in the *abhyasa* side of the chariot of sadhana.

On the *vairagya* side meditation is key to mental and emotional purification and to the creation of detachment, at least partially through its role in producing visual-kinesthetic dissociation.

In the Himalayan Tradition meditation is taught as a method. But it is also induced as an internal state through transmission and initiation. Mantra yoga is the starting point, including initiation into an individualized personal or Guru mantra. In addition to japa, the student learns to work with the mantra using the breath, particularly the spinal breath or *sumeru* breathing, as well as with the chakras. The *sumeru* breathing is a key practice for the application of *sushumna*, the opening of the flow of prana in the central *nadi* or channel in the spinal cord at the subtle level. With the opening of *sushumna* the way is clear for the raising of the kundalini energy. Swami Rama used to say with a smile that the process of enlightenment was actually quite simple. First you learn to apply *sushumna*. Then you raise the kundalini through that channel, chakra by chakra until it unites in Self-Realization in *sahasrara*.

The Still One-Pointed Mind

One could take the position that meditation cannot be taught! In fact what is taught is concentration or *dharana* and supportive states such as *pratyahara* or withdrawal of the senses. When concentration on the mantra becomes sufficiently one-pointed and stable then the state of meditation ensues spontaneously with the effortless and uninterrupted flow of the single thought towards its object. The mind field becomes coherent in the same way that a laser is coherent relative to diffuse ambient light. The mental force generated is very powerful. It can penetrate the unconscious mind and awaken the deeper forces of the personality.

Aside from its single content, the object of concentration, the concentrated mind is still. When the student learns to take the mantra into the Silence then the mind is not empty even though it is silent and still. At this point the effulgence of the Centre of Consciousness will gradually begin to fill that stillness as a Presence.

Reliable access to the Centre requires some mental control in the form of stillness of the mind. If one can carry some measure of that stillness in the background of the mind in the midst of life then the Centre can also be accessed in daily activity as well. But if the mind is turbulent with either thoughts or emotions, then access to the Centre is blocked just as surely as clouds in the sky cover the sun.

Of Maps and Methods

For a journey one needs both a map and methods for travelling. In the case of the spiritual journey the map comes from the philosophy explicated in the texts of the Tradition and in the teachings. In this case method refers to the practices of spiritual *sadhana*. Without the practices the journey cannot occur; without the maps one cannot understand the experiences on the way.

In the first part of the book we outline several maps that we have found useful for our own journey. They will make the material in the remaining sutras more understandable by creating a philosophical context for the teachings.

These maps include such things as an integrated discussion of the *yamas* and *niyamas* which are the moral precepts essential to Raja Yoga; classification of the various yogas; practical models of the personality and of the mind; and some models deriving from recent research in the physiology of host resistance.

You will find a discussion of how the mind models reality from sensory input to create your experience of the world. These models of the world or cognitive paradigms are important for understanding the perennial wisdom, particularly how Consciousness becomes bound as the limited ego. These paradigms are the maps that underlie the process of achieving nonattachment.

Cognitive maps have both structure and content. Both create the beliefs and values that determine our experience of reality as well as our behaviour and actions. Modern psychology has many effective interventions for altering the structure and content of cognitive paradigms in order to change beliefs and values. The resulting shifts in one's subjective experience of reality create new actions and behaviours. Psychology can now make important contributions to mental and emotional purification and to the creation of nonattachment.

Changing values and beliefs to realign one's mental structure to the Centre of Consciousness is an essential aspect of creating the *vairagya* in the chariot of *sadhana* that forms the basis of our *samahita* yoga. Swami Rama spoke many times about the importance of having a philosophy of life. The content and structure of these paradigms or models of the world make up what he referred to as a philosophy of life. A philosophy of life is another way to refer to the map needed for the spiritual journey.

The sutra format allows us to address the western tendency for students to cover material at too superficial a level. This kind of material needs to be absorbed deeply into the mind so that one's models of the world begin to change in a way that brings alignment to the Centre of Consciousness.

In the contemplative of process of Jnana Yoga the first step, *shravana*, refers to the intake of the material by listening to lectures or tapes, or by reading books and texts. Often this is as far as students get, acknowledging that at least the material was covered. But at this level the material is not well understood, not integrated with one's own philosophy, and at best is just memorized. This can lead to the practices becoming a ritual and the teachings becoming a rigid cult, a set of rules to be slavishly followed. Students cannot distinguish the true teachings from all the trappings such as religion, Indian culture and the social culture that has grown up around yoga itself. Nor can students discern the unity of the true teachings in other expressions of spirituality. Students begin to argue that theirs is the only way. Wearing saffron or an asana suit does not make a yogi (Swami Muktibodhananda Saraswati, 1985, p160). One needs the spirit of the law rather than the letter of the law, to use an analogy.

But you should not mistake the intent of these statements to indicate that discipline is not needed. If you are going to learn yoga, find authentic material and learn the methods correctly. Master them and always use them with awareness. This is discipline as opposed to habit and ritual.

Superficial understanding also can lead to misinterpretation and misunderstandings of the teachings and of the inner experiences. This situation eventually can result in corruption of the teachings, with unauthentic and incorrect material being given to students.

To create the change that brings alignment with the Centre one must take the learning process much deeper. Astute students should always question the authenticity of spiritual teachings. Swami Rama emphasized the importance of asking discerning questions of the master. The exigencies of the spiritual path are such that one should be sure about and have faith in the authenticity of the teachings and of the teacher in order to carry the momentum of the practice until some realization is achieved. Alignment with the Centre of Consciousness is essential to be able to make this judgment. When it is well established, the intuition from the Centre will allow students to be able to judge the authenticity of any teaching that is offered beyond just an appeal to authority.

But unfortunately few students move beyond the initial stage of *shravana*. They become addicted to seminars, speakers, tapes and books and never seem to receive fulfillment or to achieve spiritual movement. One sees this phenomenon in other fields such as psychology or personal growth. Individuals are always enthusiastically attending the "seminar of the day". Yet in spite of many years spent in the pursuit of the "latest," they never seem to resolve their personality issues.

To go the next step deeper it is important to ponder and rethink the teachings through a process of contemplation that brings a deep and full understanding of the material and begins to integrate it with one's existing philosophy. This is the step of *manana* in Jnana Yoga. The material is always on the mind, an ongoing contemplation, almost like an obsessive rumination. The mind turns it over and over at every opportunity, questioning, wondering, analysing - but always with a sense of inner expectation and listening to the Centre for Its response. One-pointedness of mind honed by concentration and meditation aids the process enormously. The concepts take shape at deeper and deeper levels, like a kind of mental digestion. And then suddenly there may come a full intuitive gestalt into the mind from the Centre, a fully born realization. To receive wisdom one must ask; this is how one asks. Casual curiosity receives no response. There must be a deep and one-pointed desire for Truth.

How often, if ever, do students sit and contemplate a single sutra from a text like the Gita, for an extended time? In these days of hurry (Swamiji used to call it "hurry, worry and curry"!), one tries to do more and more in less time. While this produces breadth, it does not produce depth. And depth is what is required for working with the Centre of Consciousness. It is better to select the very few best texts and teachings and plough them deep. In fact, when the Centre is sufficiently awakened It will provide intuitive guidance in this regard. Let the Centre of Consciousness choose your reading - it substantially cuts down on the size of the pile of books!

There comes a time when books and studying have to be left behind. "When a swami renounces the world, he often acquires the desire for learning. He learns this thing and that, studies of this book and that. Finally he finds that even the desire for learning is an obstacle for the highest attainment." (Swami Rama, 1999b). Although useful at first, the desire for information and knowledge is still just another desire. As long as you have any desires, you will not be at peace. "If you attain that center within with the help of meditation, then you will have peace of mind." (Swami Rama, 1999b). Eventually you must trade collecting "information about", which we call knowledge in the West, for direct knowing or realization from the Centre of Consciousness.

To achieve this you must go further even than the intellectual process of *manana* to the next stage of *nididhyasana* where one meditates deeply on this mentally digested truth until its intuitive realization is achieved - the final step of *sakshatkara*. Here the concentrated sutra format becomes like a probe that stimulates the student's own intuitions - like a key that unlocks the intuitive flow from the Centre of Consciousness. Like anything else in the personality the more one uses this access the finer and better it becomes as a guide to *sadhana* and to life. Students discover that Truth is an aspect of Being. And the only thing which you can take with you at the time of death is your state of being. You will have to leave your information, however cleverly contrived and integrated, behind.

With awareness anchored in the Centre of Consciousness and a practical philosophy of life you can stand on your own two feet and be independent. There comes a time when you will need no external teacher; the Inner Teacher will be your Guide to the end. You will be able to walk the path fearlessly. No one can carry you to the mountain top. You can be guided, but eventually you must climb to the peak yourself to achieve complete mastery. This is not like the dentist whose office carried the sign, "we cater to cowards." Swami Rama would say that the Himalayan Tradition is a path of mastership and is for the courageous. One learns from experience that fears are dissolved in the love flowing from the Centre of Consciousness.

Life and Death

You may be surprised to find material in this book on death. The major theme of the text is the integration of yoga and the influence of the Centre of Consciousness into daily life. Death is as much a part of life as birth. Swami Rama used to describe life as a book in progress with no beginning and no ending. Facing death forces people to confront life's ultimate questions and to begin the spiritual search. We strongly recommend that you study Swami Rama's last book entitled *Sacred Journey, Living Purposefully and Dying Gracefully* (1996) for a profound study of living and dying within the context of the *Kathopanishad*.

As health professionals we have always been puzzled at how few individuals ever really address these key issues in life, and at how most die and never ask what it was all about. Yoga brings important wisdom to this phase of life that is practical and that reaches far beyond mere academics or philosophy. It relates aspects of death to initiation and to the role of sleep and meditation as models of the dying process. The practices produce, by degrees, control over the process of dying and develop the ability to drop the body consciously.

The Centre of Consciousness and the mantram play a key role at the transition of death. But for them to operate effectively they must be cultivated in living until they are natural and spontaneous. Since one can never know when death may arrive (unless one is a very advanced adept), one should undertake the art of impeccable living - to live life as a warrior as though every day was the last. Most of us can rise to respond to an acute crisis. But when the crisis becomes ongoing and chronic, then the real testing begins. It is how the little details of each day are handled rather than the occasional big crises, that accumulate to influence the final result.

The philosophy of the Himalayan Tradition is very clear: you die as you have lived. The preparation for a good death is a good life. The time to prepare is now, daily.

Individuals who face the challenge of fatal or chronic severe disease know very well how to live with gratitude and appreciation in the moment, one day at a time. Life is full of unexpected happenings, ninety degree turns that can totally shift the momentum and direction of living. As one satirist put it, "Life's uncertain; have dessert first!" So live life absorbed in the Centre of Consciousness and you will die into the Centre of Consciousness with the Inner Teacher as your Guide.

Practical Matters

We would like this text to be practical. We have explained how the sutra format can help to do this by facilitating contemplative study. We have noted the role that repetition plays throughout the text by allowing the student to explore a truth or concept from many aspects to deepen understanding. We have also indicated the importance of the East-West synthesis of science and mysticism which you will also find throughout the text. This harmonizes with Swami Rama's own mission of bridging East and West given to him by his own Guru.

This introduction has provided a global map and set a general context for the text. The sutras themselves are divided into five sections. Section I on Foundation addresses the nature of the Centre of Consciousness, the meaning of qualification, and basic models related to the personality. After laying this foundation by providing the maps for the journey, section II addresses the inner mystical experience of the awakening of the Centre of Consciousness and the Inner Teacher so that you, the reader, are clear about what the experience is about and how to recognize it. Once the Centre opens and teaching begins there is a first curriculum presented to the disciple. This is the subject of section III. Section IV now addresses the obtaining of spiritual devotion, the subject of transpersonal visioning and the role of meditation. With section V comes an appreciation of the blessing and then of the opportunity afforded by the opening of the Centre, with a final summary of the essential path.

Particularly in the section on the first curriculum, you will find that the commentary for many of the sutras begins with a short list headed "Keys for Contemplation". The points in the list are like sub or secondary sutras that summarize the key points in the commentary to follow in order to facilitate study and contemplation. Imagine them to be like the summary points on a slide or overhead used as a visual aid for a lecture.

An extensive bibliography of references is provided to aid the student who may wish to pursue aspects of the text in more depth. For readers who may not be familiar with academic citations, these are noted in the text by brackets with first author and year of publication, for example, (Jones, 1998). The full citations are then arranged alphabetically by first author and year in the bibliography. A short glossary of Sanskrit terms is given for reference. It is not easy to index a text of sutras. The table of contents serves as a listing and index to the sutras themselves, and we have added a short index at the end of the book as well. We encourage you to pursue the explanatory endnotes for a deeper discussion of some of the sutras. These are marked by numbers in the text, such as (1).

Finally, we ask one thing of you, the reader. You may have difficulty with some of the material to be presented, either in comprehension or in acceptance. Rather than dismissing the concepts we urge you to take them into that special place in your mind where you keep things yet to be integrated and just hang them up there for now. One day you will be prompted to take them down off the hook and to try them on again. You may be surprised to find that now they fit.

Acknowledgements

We gratefully acknowledge the love and guidance of the late H.H. Sri Swami Rama to whom this book is dedicated. To Swami Veda Bharati who shares the dedication we give special thanks for teaching and guidance over so many years, and who provided the inspiration to write. We have benefited by the influence of so many students and disciples from the Himalayan Tradition whose inspiration and wisdom is reflected in the pages of this book. We especially acknowledge Swami Hariharanada, Pandit Rajmani Tigunait, Pandit Harishankar Dabral, Dr. Aruna Bhargava, Professor Vinay Bourai, Dr. Rolf and Mary-Gail Sovik, and Dr. Shiv and Savitri Jugdeo. We offer special thanks to those who have given us of their time and wisdom or who have acted as reviewers, especially Mayanne Krech, Sarah and Andrew Wilson, and MaLa Sahan. To our many colleagues of the Foothills Yoga Society and to other devotees of yoga in Calgary, Alberta and Canada who have influenced us we express appreciation for learning and support. And our family, Paul and Leslie Jerry and Marc and Marnie Jerry - fellow travellers on the Path - we acknowledge specially.

I FOUNDATION

Peace be in heavens
Peace be in skies
Peace be on earth
May the waters flow peacefully
May the herbs and shrubs grow peacefully
May all the divine powers bring us peace
The supreme Brahman is peace
May all be at peace
Peace and only peace
And may that peace come to us all
AUM
Shantih, shantih, shantih
Peace, peace, peace

(Swami Veda Bharati, Superconscious Meditation, Tape 2106)

The Centre of Consciousness

1. Now begins instruction on how to work with the Centre of Consciousness.

These first three sections describing the *Centre of Consciousness*, *Qualification* and *Personality*, introduce the main text which starts at Section II - *Mystical Experience of the Centre of Consciousness*. They sketch a context or background of core knowledge, an intellectual map of key concepts as a foundation on which the discussions in Section II can rest.

In classical Sanskrit texts, commentaries on sutras often begin with the word, *atha*, or "now". The word is used in the sense of a starting point within a longer ongoing process. The word *anantarya* (transition in a sequence) may also be used (Arya, 1986). Like the modern educational process which can spread over decades for a highly specialized professional such as a specialist physician, the process of spiritual unfoldment stretches over life times. In the educational system there are major transitions between levels of schooling: from public to high school; from high school to university; from undergraduate to graduate studies; or from graduate to post graduate work. Then there are minor transitions from academic year to year (each even with different preceptors!), within major blocks of study, and transitions between subjects at the beginning and ending of specific courses of study.

So it is on the Spiritual Path. There are sign posts to mark the different phases of the journey. Some are minor markers to indicate progress. Others are prominent to mark major transitions and stages along the Path that take the pilgrim into entirely new aspects of spiritual unfoldment. To step across the threshold of one of these major transitions is to be reborn into an expanded and entirely new *weltanschauung* (world view). The word *atha*, "now", marks one of these major transitions and also implies qualification (*adhikara*). Having completed all that is gone before, the aspirant has been tested and is now qualified to begin the next step of the Path. This is meant in the same way that a student has completed the four or five years of high school, for example, has passed the final examinations, has passed the entry examinations to university, and now is qualified, is ready to begin university work (a very major transition in every way as those who have experienced it will attest!).

Why do we speak here of a major transition on the Path? The opening of the Centre of Consciousness within the student's inner subjective experience is a major development that introduces significant qualitative changes in subjective experience. It creates a turning point for the student's level of commitment to the Spiritual Path - a point from which there can be no return.

2. *The Centre of Consciousness is the Inner Teacher, the Inner Guru.*

What is the Centre of Consciousness? Our spiritual preceptor, the late H. H. Sri Swami Rama, described it simply as the core or centre of one's being from which consciousness flows in various degrees and grades.

Each of us has a divine core, a soul, called the Atman, or Self. We each carry a fragment of God within us. The task of the Spiritual Path is Self-Realization, to become aware of our spiritual nature within and to express it fully. The Centre of Consciousness is one of the first manifestations of Spirit, of spirituality, or of spiritual consciousness, as distinct from ordinary thoughts, feelings and sensations that make up our normal waking experience. This first manifestation is called the Inner Teacher or Inner Guru. It has many names in many traditions.

It is a radically new aspect of consciousness in the sense that the acquisition of sight would be to the experience of someone born blind. Those who have vision can share that experience in ways that someone who is blind can only imagine. Likewise, those who know the Centre can recognize and communicate that experience with others who know. But the experience cannot be imagined by or communicated in language to someone who yet does not know. It is a secret that once revealed remains a secret.

This kind of experiential direct knowing is what is referred to in the texts frequently as Knowledge. It is not knowledge as we understand it in the West in the sense of intellectual information or understanding about something. For imagination, conceptualization and language are faculties of the intellect whose constructions, however creative or bizarre, can only be based on reorganizations and transformations of elements taken from what is already known, from past experience. They cannot construct a radically and qualitatively new inner experience. The effect must always proceed from the cause; the effect is inherent in the cause. The tendency of Western science to try to explain such things as "emergent properties" of what went before, of something simpler, does not apply here.

> "It is important to remember that the consciousness, the Atman or the Self, does not actually evolve. There is no evolution of the Atman, or soul. By the practice of (Yoga) we do not actually evolve; it is a process of involution. It is not true to say that our souls have evolved from the primitive state to our present developed state. The supreme existence, or the soul, is the same as it was thousands of years ago. It does not undergo a change. The only difference is that our lower self or the individualized self becomes aware of that supreme form slowly, step-by-step.
>
> When we turn our minds from the outer world to the inner world, we come to know that there is an infinite facet of existence in us which can only be experienced in samadhi. It is not approachable through the intellect, therefore a sadhana like the eight rungs of Raja Yoga is required."
> Swami Satyananda Saraswati (1989), pp 226-227.

3. It is awakened through the grace of one's Spiritual Preceptor by initiation.

4. The Spiritual Preceptor is a messenger whose task is to deliver the wisdom of the sages of the Himalayan Tradition.

5. His or her task is also to introduce the qualified student to the teacher within.

Our Gurudev, Sri Swami Rama, described his role with these words, "I am a messenger, delivering the wisdom of the Himalayan Sages of my Tradition. My job is to introduce you to the Teacher within."

The Himalayan Tradition is an initiatory Tradition. The essence of the definition of a guru in the Himalayan Tradition is one can give *shaktipat*, higher spiritual initiations that involve the transmission of spiritual energy (*shakti*) at

36 Sutras of the Inner Teacher

various levels and intensities according to the capacity and qualification of the student to receive.

The properly initiated student who begins to realize the Centre within will learn that the Centre and his or her guru or external master are one and the same in consciousness. To have that Centre opened into awareness is to have one's own "pocket guru" within, so to speak; to move into having continuous access to the love, guidance and wisdom of the master through inner access, regardless of where the master may be located physically. Indeed, a student with this inner contact may spend very little time with the master physically, but remain in continuous inner contact. A key goal of the training at this point on the Path is to strengthen that inner contact so that it becomes effective. Such a contact is, in effect, a continuous link with one's own spiritual Self, rather than some kind of hypnotic mind control. This is the ultimate in pedagogy!

The Bhagavad Gita is a text par excellence that describes this interaction between the consciousness of the qualified disciple, Arjuna, and the Inner Teacher, Krishna, who guides him on the battlefield of life. The teachings in this text show the depth and quality of the practical spiritual guidance that can flow to the disciple from within as he or she negotiates daily life.

> *"7. My will is paralyzed, and I am utterly confused. Tell me which is the better path for me. Let me be your disciple. I have fallen at your feet; give me instruction.*
>
> Arjuna tells Sri Krishna, "I am your disciple. Now be my teacher and instruct me." In the Orthodox Hindu tradition, until we ask the teacher to be our guru, showing our readiness to receive his guidance on the path of meditation, he does not offer to do this for us. ...The word guru means 'one who is heavy,' so heavy that he can never be shaken. A guru is a person who is so deeply established within himself that no force on earth can affect the complete love he feels for everyone. If you curse him, he will bless you; if you harm him, he will serve you; and if you exploit him, he will become your benefactor. It is good for us to remember that the guru, the spiritual teacher, is in everyone of us. All that another person can do is to make us aware of the teacher within ourselves. The outer teacher makes us aware of the teacher within, and to the extent we can be loyal to the outer teacher, we are being loyal to ourselves, to our Atman. ...
>
> ... When the disciples love the guru, it is this love that unifies their consciousness. At the time when we are ready for it, the spiritual teacher will step aside to show us that all the love we have been giving him has been directed to our own Atman. ... it is in order to unify the consciousness of the disciple that the relationship exists. ...

❈

> ... If you are prepared to undertake the long journey, the teacher will give you the map and all necessary instructions, but you have got to do the travelling yourself. That the teacher cannot provide. The purpose of visiting a spiritual teacher is to be reminded that there is a destination, there is a supreme goal in life, and we all have the innate capacity to undertake the journey. When people used to sit in the presence of Sri Ramana Maharshi and praise him, he would just smile as if to say, "There is no Sri Ramana Maharshi. I am just a little keyhole through which, when you fix your eye with complete concentration, you can see the beckoning, irresistible vision of the Lord."
>
> Bhagavad Gita II.7 (Easwaran, 1975, pp 54-55)

But in the choice of a spiritual teacher and master much discrimination is required. It is said that the student receives the kind of teacher he or she deserves. Truly enlightened beings are rare enough on the planet, but good students are even rarer. We searched for many years to find a live and authentic tradition of yoga. Regrettably so much of what is presented in the bookstore and the lecture hall in the West simply does not qualify. Fortunately the Centre of Consciousness and initiation will always guide the sincere student back to his or her tradition and master in any given lifetime. Yogananda would often talk about meeting friends from other lives. Once the karma of a particular lifetime has been worked through the student will be ready to pick up the spiritual journey from where he or she left off in the last lifetime. The student will be led back to the Path through a series of synchronicities triggered by the intent to search. The master will appear at the appropriate time. But the external master is only a guide. The traveller on the Path may be in the company of many others outside, but ultimately he or she makes the journey within alone with the Inner Teacher.

> "As a young man during the decades following World War II, I became passionately engaged in a search for living exemplars of spiritual realization. Venturing far and wide, I sought out, in addition to the dervishes, Hindu yogis and rishis, as well as Buddhist and Christian monks. Of the many ascetics I encountered on this quest, most, in my estimation, ultimately failed to pass the test of authenticity. Some, it seemed, derived satisfaction from exercising power over seekers; others were very skilled in the art of sophisticated trickery - and little else - while still others became renowned simply because they attracted increasingly larger audiences. Yet the absence of true mystical depth on the part of so many only served to make my encounters with the rare beings of true enlightenment that much more powerful. In their presence I felt uplifted, as if I were "walking on air." The effects of their realization upon others was palpable; their inner sovereignty was so great that they were able to help people gain their self-confidence."
>
> Pir Vilayat Inayat Khan, 1999, p67

When you have had the privilege of meeting a realized master and receiving his or her *darshan* you will experience that feeling of inner divine upliftment flowering in and around you. Your discrimination makes a giant leap forward. Now it will be much simpler for you to distinguish authentic teaching and guidance through this gift of discernment which comes from the master to the student.

Adhikara: Qualification

6. The Centre of Consciousness awakens only in the qualified student.

Keys to Contemplation

- **Defining qualification as the six treasures.**
- **Prerequisites to imparting a teaching.**
- **Rejuvenation of the personality.**

In the first sutra we touched upon the idea of qualification (*adhikara*) when we considered the word "now" (*atha*). In traditional texts the word "now" expresses either *anantarya* (transition in a sequence) or *adhikara* (referring to the authority of the teacher or a student's fulfillment of qualification, or simply a statement of commencement) (Arya, 1986, p67).

What do we mean by qualified? The philosophical texts of Vedanta, especially, define a qualified student as one who has practised the "six treasures" (*shat-sampat*) (Arya, 1986):

shama	Mental quietude and control of the passions; a gentle and peaceful temperament.
dama	Restraint of the five senses (hearing, touch, sight, taste and smell) as well as the five active senses (speech from the mouth; grasping by the hands; locomotion by the feet; evacuation from the anus; and the genitals for generation). It also includes restraint of the four internal organs (*ahamkara* or the ego; *chitta* or the memory; *buddhi*, the understanding; and *manas*, cognition) There is control of thoughts, desires and emotions so that the eyes and ears are not darting about restlessly with the hands and feet in constant motion from nervous energy.
uparati	Complete cessation of the perceiving and acting faculty. A withdrawal from desires and worldly possessions, yet

	remaining involved, performing immediate duties lovingly and perfectly without seeking their fruits.
titiksha	Patience and the power to endure the pairs of opposites like extremes of heat and cold, joy and sorrow, honour and abuse, loss and gain, etc. Fortitude, forbearance, the ability to bear insult and discomfort without complaining or feeling that one is suppressing one's natural urges or "rights".
samadhana	Continual concentration of the mind. Harmony and freedom from conflict within oneself as well as the ability to resolve conflict in one's external environment and relationships.
shraddha	Faith, humility, surrender; conviction and devotion that one is on the right path and has the right guru who is competent to lead one to enlightenment.

" ... then, pacified, controlled, having withdrawn,
forbearing, harmonized, one should see the Self in the
self."
                       Brihadaranyaka Upanishad IV.4.23

In the Tradition there are preparations that are prerequisites to imparting a teaching:
• how seriously a student applies himself or herself and the kinds of questions he or she raises;
• the quality and extent of practice - ascetic observances and purifications, and the
• preparation of the body.

Nowadays the latter would include lifestyle issues such as exercise, diet, supplements, etc., in addition to the standard regimen of yoga *sadhana*. In the past it would have included the ancient medical science of *ayurveda* which prescribed a process for rejuvenation of the body. The practices were very complex, and included internal purifications, diet, herbs, and compounds containing mercury, sulfur and gold. These *rasayanas* or rejuvenation practices intended an alteration of body chemistry to support protracted periods of *samadhi* and to strengthen the body for strenuous practices. When the *kundalini* is raised the spiritual energy produces an actual slow physical transformation of biology so that it can eventually hold and express the full force of the Centre of Consciousness, the Self, the Atman, the soul. The analogy is given of putting very high voltage through a wire that has not the capacity to handle it, and it burns up. The capacity of the wire is raised by purifying it through removing impurities in the metal that produce the resistance and heat. A well-known example of the exigencies that such a process can produce in an unprepared aspirant is graphically described in the writings of Gopi Krishna (1974).

The biology of the physical body functions around a homeostatic principle. The set points for homeostasis in health are not static, but the result of a dynamic process consisting of the integrated movement of many factors in response to the influence of both the internal and external environments. The process is one of continuous movement towards the equilibrium point, and some use the term homeodynamic rather than homeostatic to emphasize this ceaseless activity. Dysfunction and disease can be considered to be a breakdown in this homeostasis, while health can be defined in terms of balance and stable equilibrium. Vital functions such as respiration, blood pressure or heart rate, and biochemical parameters in health are all held within precise and narrow limits. The phenomenon would remind one of the tall inflated balloons in the shape of a clown made for children. The feet are weighted to make the clown stand upright in such a way that no matter how hard the child hits it, the clown pops right back up to its standing equilibrium position. The transformative effects of *sadhana* mentioned above address not just the restoration of homeostasis within the personality with the creation of health, but also something much more fundamental - the raising of the vibratory level of the homeostatic set point itself.

There are many stories surrounding the purity of the physical vehicle of a master and its resistance to disease and decay. After his *mahasamadhi* the dead physical body of Paramahansa Yogananda (1983) showed no visual signs of decay even after 20 days in the mortuary.

The point is that in addition to moral behaviour there are deeper considerations of qualification here about the readiness of biology to contain the higher energies of advanced spiritual realization.

In the Tantric tradition an analogous set of qualifications exist (Johari, 1986). The first six give control over one's animal or biological nature and include:

daksha	intelligence
jitendriya	control over the senses
sarva hinsa vinirmukta	abstention from violence of any kind
shuchi	purity
astik	a belief in truth defined as *vidya* (knowledge), *veda* (body

of knowledge) and God.

The other qualifications in Tantra are the same six treasures of Vedanta listed above. It is suggested that they coordinate the various levels of the brain such as the brain stem, R-complex and cerebral cortex. The brain stem is the oldest part of the brain phylogenetically and controls essential vegetative autonomic activities like respiration as well as cardiovascular functions like heart rate and blood pressure.

With evolutionary progress comes Paul MacLean's R-complex (1984; Papez, 1937) which caps the brain stem and is the seat of aggression, ritual, territoriality and social hierarchy. This is, in turn, surmounted by the limbic system which is the source of moods and emotions as well as concern and care for the young. Finally comes the most recently evolved outer covering of the brain, the cerebral cortex, which mediates functions such as consciousness, inspiration, abstract thinking, musical composition, reading and writing (1).

In general, purification practices are thought to energize the body and to create electrochemical balance. Pranayama stimulates the brain stem, while ritual and discipline are thought to stimulate the R-complex (Johari, 1986). *Dhyana* including mantra and japa as well as visualization stimulate the cerebral cortex.

It is proposed that these six treasures coordinate all of these functioning levels of the brain in all three states of waking, dreaming and deep sleep. They lead the aspirant to superconsciousness or *turiya*.

7. Strict commitment to moral behaviour is assumed, both for qualification and even after the awakening of the Centre of Consciousness.

8. Otherwise there is risk of a fall.

Keys to Contemplation

- **Moral behaviour is assumed.**
- **Know them by their actions.**
- **Increasing refinement of the standard of right speech and action.**
- **Guidance of the Centre of Consciousness is essential.**

These two sutras are of paramount importance and underlie the basis of some of the material that will be covered in the section on curriculum below. In the Gita (14:21) Krishna responds in great detail about the behaviour of an enlightened being. How are we to judge whether an individual is enlightened? The answer is actually straightforward: "Ye shall know them by their fruits." (Matthew 7: 16). In more modern language, they walk their talk!

If someone claims that he is enlightened then the would-be student should beware. Enlightened behaviour is many things - wise, loving, kind, etc. - but one thing it always is, is moral. The morality flows in speech and action naturally and spontaneously from such a being because it is the result of his or her egoless nature. Morality is so fundamental that it is assumed as a prerequisite at this stage of the path.

The opening of the Centre of Consciousness makes right speech and right action easier, but the aspirant must still be on guard. Although to some measure advanced, the process of transformation by *sadhana* is not yet complete. It is still possible for such a one to fall, even after this degree of achievement.

At this level the temptations do not come in obvious form like murder or theft. Such a one has no difficulty avoiding these. The ego is clever. It presents the challenges in very subtle ways such as issues of integrity, fairness and justice, ambition, co-dependencies in relationships, sexuality disguised as love and romance, conflicting personal agendas, ethics in handling resources and money, unwitting exploitation of helpers, issues around power and control, fame and reputation, secrecy (knowledge withheld is power), etc.

> "For these vices of the ordinary man pass through a subtle transformation and reappear with changed aspect in the heart of the disciple.
> ... the pure artist who works for the love of his work is sometimes more firmly planted on the right road than the occultist, who fancies he has removed his interest from self, but who has in reality only enlarged the limits of experience and desire, and transferred his interest to the things which concern his larger span of life."
> Collins, 1976, p18

It takes increasing discrimination by the aspirant to work through these challenges with true understanding, for they all have the potential to produce negative karma. What is moral for one individual in one context may not be for another in a different context. The process is relative in the sense that there is an increasingly refined standard applied as the student progresses. Here the guidance of the Centre of Consciousness in everyday life becomes essential.

❁

9. *The restraints (yamas) and observances (niyamas) of Raja Yoga form the core of morality.*

The *yamas* and the *niyamas* should be well-known to any serious student of yoga. These "ten commandments" of yoga have analogies in other traditions, for example, the ten commandments in the Christian Bible. They constitute respectively the first two rungs on the ladder of Patanjali's Ashtanga or Raja Yoga (Aranya, 1981), which is the foundation of the Himalayan Tradition.

Much lip service is given to them by yoga teachers, but once enunciated - often in but a single class - they are left behind for more challenging and interesting things like hatha or pranayama. Perhaps in the West this cursory treatment is in part due to our discomfort with moral precepts in our materialistic culture where only visible results relevant to the bottom line matter. Or perhaps it is because some research is needed on how to teach them effectively in a way that allows the student to work with them over a prolonged period to integrate these attitudes into daily life and living.

One should be very clear what is meant here. Although we use words like "moral" or "ethics", we do not intend them in any religious or philosophical sense. This is not about "being a nice person"; not about likeability, avoiding conflict, and not about "not rocking the boat." It is also not about discovering Truth. Truth is already known. It is about hearing what is True and then incorporating that Truth, saturating the whole personality with it, thereby transforming its structure to remove mental objectors and ignorance until a structure is created that is capable of holding Spirit for direct realization. It is about changing one's pictures of reality so that one's mental structure is realigned with these Truths. One purifies by taking out the resistance, so that the mind can become a fit vessel to receive the higher energies of Spirit.

It is not our intention to discuss the *yamas* and *niyamas* in detail here. But we would like to offer a way to think of them in a more integrated manner other than as a "laundry list" of do's and don'ts as they are usually presented. The schema is summarized in Figure 1: "Yoga in Daily Life: Meditation in Action". Initially one works with these attitudes as practices. In the enlightened master these attitudes are spontaneous. They are a natural state of being and hence are totally trustworthy. They are the means of "raising life to the level of your meditation" as so eloquently phrased by Swami Veda Bharati.

44 Sutras of the Inner Teacher

10. Ahimsa (non-injury), satya (truthfulness), asteya (non-stealing), brahmacharya (continence) and aparigraha (non-possessiveness) are the yamas (restraints).

The five *yamas* work with the outer world: avoid doing these things so as not to make trouble for others and for yourself (Figure 1, p45). They deal with external context, with the environment, and specifically with relationships. Swami Rama said often that life is relationships; relationships are the warp and woof of daily life and living.

Non-injury or non-violence is the core of the *yamas*. To be given the real power of mastership an adept must become wholly harmless in every way: "Let no living being fear me." Although little has been written about the *yamas* and *niyamas*, with the possible exception of *brahmacharya*, perhaps most has been said about non-violence. Gandhi's studies of *satygraha* and non-violence are classic and should be studied by the sincere student.

Related to non-violence is truthfulness. The adept must become not only harmless but transparent. Both qualities arise from coherence of the personality through the elimination of inner conflict through alignment of the personality with the Centre of Consciousness. These qualities come first from the conquest of fear, of duality. As long as there is a perception of an "other", then the issue of who or what is in control - me or the "other"- arises. Swami Rama so often urged his students and disciples to learn to be fearless. From fear flows anger and internal conflict. From attachment comes self-identified infatuation and involvement leading to pain, suffering and grief. Ultimately transparency flows from non-attachment.

Brahmacharya is often presented in terms of celibacy, but its meaning is much broader. It means moderation and continence in all things of the senses.

> "One should maintain a balance in the normal behavioral pattern of emotion, consciousness or energy ... [leading] to the expansions of our inner faculties. This leads to a developed awareness of the Self, which is brahmacharya.
>
> Brahma means supreme, divine, higher, and Acharya means knower of, or master. The absolute meaning of brahmacharya is not sensual abstinence, rather it is the merger of the individual with the higher consciousness and constantly maintaining that identity. Sexual abstinence came to be known as part of brahmacharya when evolved beings noted that passionless and desire free relationships with the opposite sex gave an insight into the transcendental awareness which is free of gross feelings.

Yoga In Daily Life
Meditation in Action

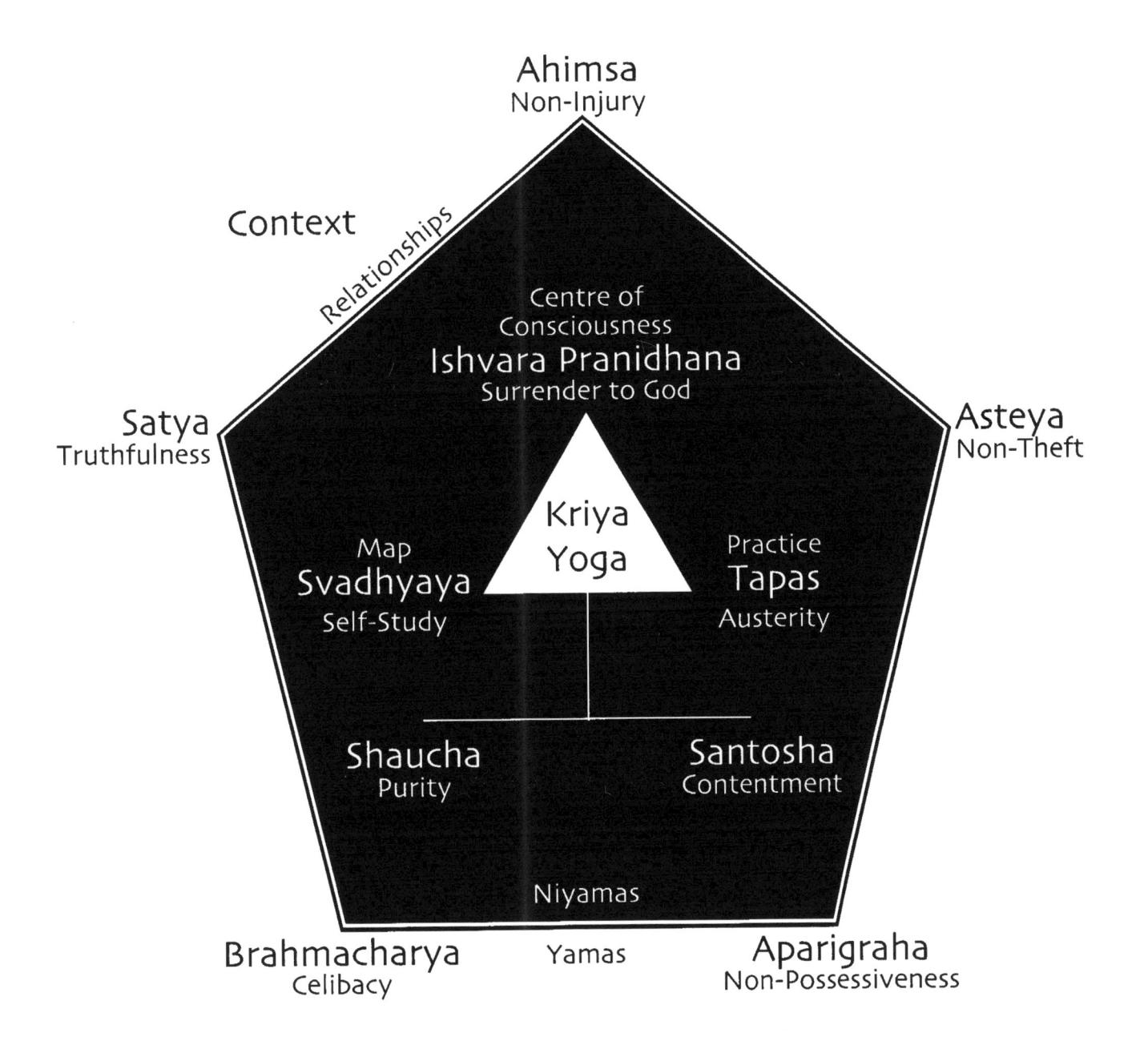

Ahimsa
Non-Injury

Context

Relationships

Satya
Truthfulness

Centre of
Consciousness
Ishvara Pranidhana
Surrender to God

Asteya
Non-Theft

Map
Svadhyaya
Self-Study

Kriya
Yoga

Practice
Tapas
Austerity

Shaucha
Purity

Santosha
Contentment

Niyamas

Brahmacharya
Celibacy

Yamas

Aparigraha
Non-Possessiveness

Raise Life to the Level of Your Meditation

Figure 1. The Yamas and Niyamas

>Therefore they said to abstain from animal passion so that the gross carnal desires evolve. Later in ignorance, man defined brahmacharya as total sensual and sexual abstinence to develop spiritual awareness."
>
>Paramahansa Niranjanananda, 1992, p71-72

The remaining two *yamas* are the result of gaining non-attachment (nonreaction in a broader sense) to all manifested objects, ranging from actions and things to thoughts and ideas.

The practice of the *yamas* smooths relationships in life in addition to producing right action. One no longer commits actions that will bring unpleasant consequences to complicate life, and to disturb the inner balance and equanimity produced by meditation. In being loving, kind and compassionate to life, it will reflect love, kindness and compassion back to you. For your thoughts, speech and action attract their like. It is in this way that you raise life to the level of your meditation.

Although we have talked here about transparency and harmlessness we do not wish to imply that the result is an anemic personality with all of the qualities of a door mat that everyone tramps on with impunity. Swami Rama had a charismatic and, at times, overpowering personality that radiated creativity, fearlessness and love. He was the very antithesis of a door mat! He could display a full emotional range as the situation required from the softest gentleness to hurricane force. But he did so with total control and non-attachment.

Yoga is not about destroying the ego nor is it about suppressing emotional expression as students often are taught. Emotional tone colours life in the way that harmony colours music. What must be unlearned is emotional reactivity, which is a complete loss of control and loss of inner equanimity that sunders the link with Spirit, leading the personality to unfortunate and impulsive speech and action. Swamiji once challenged us that it was one thing never to be angry, but it was something much more to learn how to use anger appropriately without losing inner equilibrium, without getting caught up in it. There is a story often told in the Tradition that makes the point.

Once a sage was travelling through a village in India. The villagers summoned his help to deal with an aggressive cobra that had all of them terrified of being bitten. The sage found the snake and admonished it for such behaviour, saying he expected it to have changed its ways when next he visited. The cobra expressed sorrow for its aggressive behaviour and promised to reform. Indeed it became the model of gentleness, and soon even the children of the village handled and played with it fearlessly. But with the loss of fear their play became careless and rough, and the villagers began to be unkind to it.

Some years later the sage again visited the village and the villagers thanked him for having solved the problem with the snake. The sage went to find the snake, but was horrified to see that it had been badly abused and was broken and bruised. When asked what had happened the snake replied that it had done its best to follow the sages's request that it not bite anyone no matter what the provocation. "Sir, I have followed your command to the letter and look what it has brought me. It is all your fault!" To which the sage replied, "Yes, I told you not to bite anyone, but I didn't tell you not to hiss!"

11. Shaucha (purity of body and mind), santosha (contentment), tapas (austerity - physical and mental discipline), svadhyaya (scriptural study and mantra repetiton) and Ishvara Pranidhana (devotion, surrender to God) are the niyamas (observances).

If the *yamas* work with the outer world, the *niyamas* work with the inner (Figure 1, p45). Three of them make up the practice of Kriya Yoga (not to be confused with the yogas of the same name from Paramahansa Yogananda or from the Bihar School of Yoga). This is a core practice at this stage of the Path that is based on purity, both mental and physical, as well as contentment - attitudes that rest in non-attachment. In short, the *yamas* help you work on your relationships to the external world, while the *niyamas* help you with transforming your inner self.

Each step in spiritual unfoldment must be integrated into the personality thoroughly before the next is taken. The energy sheaths that comprise the personality, which are reviewed below, must evolve in coordination. With each infusion of spiritual energy there is a pause, a plateau, during which the new energy is assimilated and integrated into the personality at every layer before one can go on. These dry spells can be frustrating to the student when, after seeming to make so much progress, nothing seems to be happening and progress seems stalled. But there is a great wisdom behind this. Sri Aurobindo's consort, the Mother, noted that if the sheaths surge ahead in an uncoordinated way and become out of phase, then "yogic illness" can result (The Mother, 1979). It is important that one have an integrated and balanced practice involving all the limbs of Raja Yoga.

We want to "soak" up and absorb these attitudes until they penetrate so deeply they transform the core of our models of reality. Simply hearing or reading about them is not enough. The strategy for *sadhana* in Jnana Yoga can be recommended. This sequence of *shravana, manana, nididhyasana* and *sakshatkara* is described above on page 27.

12. Tapas, svadhyaya and Ishvara pranidhana when practised together constitute Kriya Yoga, which makes up the core of yoga at this stage of the Spiritual Path by providing the practice itself, the map to guide the journey, and the goal and guidance from the Centre of Consciousness.

At this stage Kriya Yoga underlies the essential Spiritual Path. For any journey one needs a destination or goal. That is embodied in *Isvara pranidhana* or surrender to God. Here we are talking about working with the Centre of Consciousness which is a form of profound inner surrender. Besides a destination, one also needs a map for the journey. *Svadhyaya* shows the way with self-study. This includes study of the scriptures and the examples of the saints and sages that provide the map for the journey. That map must be internalized and gradually integrated into the aspirant's consciousness step by step. It must be matched with the state of development of the personality at all levels and gradual adjustments made.

Note that *svadhyaya* also includes repetition of the mantra. In this context the mantra serves as protection from the six mental enemies: *kama* - passions; *krodha* - anger; *lobha* - greed; *moha* - delusion and attachment; *Irshya* - jealousy; *mada* - pride and frenzy, including *matsarya* - small-mindedness and malice. Maintaining constant japa wards off these negative tendencies like an antidote (Arya, 1981).

All of the above concerns the map for the journey. Now we look at the process of taking the journey itself - practice, which is inherent in the word *tapas*. In this context *tapas* can be considered to represent the discipline of the practices of *sadhana*. How regular is the *sadhana*, how complete, how well integrated, of what quality? Is the time for meditation kept?

In the West the word "discipline" has a negative connotation. It is full of resistance, full of "shoulds" and "oughts". *Sadhana* is a co-creative process between the small self and Spirit that involves full transformation of the entire personality so that it can express the full magnificence of the Self in mastership. As such it needs the passion of any creative process. Living life is an art.

When we speak of discipline we rather mean the discipline of the artist, musician or writer, of the elite athlete, of the scientist, of the professional physician, of the entrepreneurial businessperson. Each of these individuals thinks nothing of dedicating 18 hours a day for well over a decade beyond basic schooling to achieve excellence in their calling. Yet in spirituality we seem to resent making a similar commitment for what is an even grander outcome. The artist or sculptor learns his technique, the concert pianist learns her scales and arpeggios, the surgeon learns his craft. All of them attack the challenge of mastering their art with passion, and once they have achieved mastery then they transcend their technology to create magnificently, whether it is art, music or healing. It is only through the control that the mastery of technique provides that a talented individual can express creatively.

There are three components here: one is achieving mastery of one's medium of expression by transcending technique; another is passion; and the third is loving the process with one-pointedness without attachment to the outcome.

The transformation of *sadhana* is approached in the same way. Turn your life inside out. Instead of your career, for example, make your *sadhana* the polestar around which your whole life revolves. Then your career, your whole life will be a moment to moment expression of it. Love your *sadhana* as you love God, for it is both your service and your worship to the Divine. Swami Rama would often say, "Sheva is my puja," service is my worship. This is true Karma Yoga.

Tapas can have a special meaning here as well. The transformation we are talking about is changing beliefs and values, changing the energetic configurations that construct our pictures of reality in the mind field, the world view that defines our ego, our self-identity, who we are and what is our experience of our world. Each change is a small death since it involves shifting our self-identity. So change like this does not come easily. *Tapas* can be a Tantric key to transmuting energy (Ballentine, 1999). It can be used to transform habitual impulses relevant to the *yamas* and *niyamas*. When an urge to act in the old way arises one consciously chooses not to express it in the old habitual way regardless of the discomfort of its urgency. Rather than suppressing or denying the urging in order to avoid experiencing its force, one intentionally observes, allows, accepts and contains the building discomfort, refusing to be moved by it, until it bursts into another channel. The use of the spinal breath in meditation prepares a basis for the energy to explode upward to a higher chakra producing exhilaration and empowerment.

13. *Ishvara Pranidhana, surrender to God, awakens with the Centre of Consciousness.*

The practice of *Ishvara pranidhana* is focal to what we mean by working with the Centre of Consciousness. The method is at once the very simplest possible, and at the same time an infinitely rich process. It is simply the art of constantly remembering the Self; practising the presence of God.

The basic stance of the disciple can be summarized by service, practice, and discipline (Arya, 1981). The most important qualification the master looks for in the disciple is that he or she should be rich in the six treasures discussed under sutra 6. The aspirant should be prepared to offer service in whatever way is needed to others, to fellow initiates and their families, and to the guru's teaching mission. One must overcome the attitudes of non-commitment and uninvolvement along with the fear of consequences resulting from getting involved. One learns not to lay down conditions for one's service and involvement.

The four attitudes called *brahma-vihara* ("frolicking in God") are cultivated: *maitri* - friendship and love towards those who are happy; *karuna* - compassion towards those who suffer; *mudita* - happiness at seeing others making spiritual progress; and *upeksha* - indifference towards the evil in others, learning to help others out of love and compassion rather than from hatred towards evil. Finally, one learns to control one's speech, which should be *hitam*, *mitam* and *priyam* - beneficial, measured, and pleasant.

Swami Rama mentioned frequently the need to master the four biological urges: food, sleep, sex and self-preservation (which today we would call stress). Much of yoga practice addresses these urges, and they operate throughout our day, influencing our behaviour profoundly. Control does not mean suppression or repression of these urges as is so often incorrectly thought. It means a conscious, choiceful, balanced and harmonious expression of these natural urges of the body. There is a fifth urge which is to be strengthened - the urge to enlightenment.

The Personality

14. *The aspirant is body, breath, mind and soul or spirit.*

Aldous Huxley described the perennial wisdom, the *Philosophia Perennis* in this way:

> *"Philosophia perennis* - the phrase was coined by Leibniz; but the thing - the metaphysic that recognizes a divine Reality substantial to the world of things and lives and minds; the psychology that finds in the soul something similar to, or even identical with, divine Reality; the ethic that places man's final end in the knowledge of the immanent and transcendent Ground of all being - the thing is immemorial and universal."
>
> Huxley, 1944

The term and others like it (prisca theologia and philosophia occulta) were used in the Renaissance in reference to esoteric wisdom originating through many ancient lineages (Faivre & Needleman, 1992). It is also used as a metaphysical description of the cosmos as constructed of layers or tiers.

> "The conception of the universe as .... ranging in hierarchical order from the meagerest kind of existents ... through 'every possible' grade up to the ens perfectissimum — has, in one form or another, been the dominant official philosophy of the larger part of civilized mankind through most of its history."
>
> Lovejoy, 1936

We raise it here to present yet another essential model for the aspirant - that of the personality as layered into *koshas* or sheaths. Both Ken Wilber (1983) and Huston Smith (1982) note that virtually all of the esoteric traditions are based on the assumption of a series of layers of being that ascend from the material world of multiplicity up to a single absolute reality. Both the macrocosm (the cosmos) and the microcosm (the personality) are stratified - a concept that is over 25 centuries old and that has its most elegant expression in Vedanta.

Based on Spinoza, Huxley formulated the perennial philosophy in three statements:

1. There is an infinite, changeless Reality beneath the world of change.
2. This same Reality lies at the core of every human personality.
3. The purpose of life is to discover and to experience this Reality: that is, to realize God while here on earth.

The essence of the perennial wisdom lies in the very causation, nature and cure of suffering in general. And we would add a fourth statement:

> 4. The interior experiments for realizing this Reality constitute the science of yoga - an unbroken oral Tradition of continuous Master-Disciple relationships for over 3,000 years. There is only one Tradition, one spiritual science, but it manifests in many forms.

This fourth statement emphasizes that yoga is the science of spirituality, and that the proper study of spirituality is the practical study of this infinite, changeless, ultimate Reality, which is the Consciousness that underlies and permeates, or lies at the core of that layered universe or personality.

Let us offer a pragmatic definition of the personality given by Swami Rama: it is simply body, breath, mind and soul. Swamiji based his entire teaching on the interconnectedness of body, breath, mind and soul. "All of the body is in the mind," he would say, "but not all of the mind is in the body." As consciousness, the soul pervades the body and mind. Body, mind and soul, yes, but why breath? The word "spirit" derives from the Latin word *spiritus*, which means breath. It soon came to also mean vital power or energy and eventually an intangible element that animates a material thing. The breath plays a key role in linking body and mind. Breath control (*pranayama*) in yoga is a very important aspect of spiritual training, much less the maintenance of health and longevity. For Swamiji yoga was the spiritual practices that awakened one's inner being, bringing mastery over body, breath and mind and the fullest enjoyment of life (Tigunait, 1998). The accomplished yogi was to have full conscious and voluntary control over every level of the personality - biochemical, biological and psychological. This is what Swamiji meant by spiritual science. He defined spiritual practices as those methods that allow the practitioner of yoga to experience these truths directly.

15. Manifested reality (the universe or the individual personality) is consciousness enrobed in energy arranged in layers within a vibrational spectrum ranging from matter through the subtle (pranic) body (which is accessed by breath), to several layers of mind.

16. These interpenetrating energy fields of higher and higher vibrational frequency constitute the personality which is suffused with consciousness emanating from the core.

Now to make use of this pragmatic model of body, breath, mind and soul, one needs to ask what is meant by the personality in the perennial wisdom. Figure 2 (p54) shows the personality according to Vedanta (Swami Rama et al, 1976a). The core is the Centre of Consciousness called the Self. It is enrobed in 5 sheaths: 3 for mind, 1 for the energy body and the outermost one for the physical body. Now clearly people are not onions in cross-section! Rather, this diagram is symbolic of interpenetrating energy fields of higher and higher vibrational frequency which are suffused with consciousness emanating from that core (Yoga Vasishtha).

In the Tantric view both the individual and the universe are perceived as Consciousness, the *Shiva* principle, enrobed in energy, the *Shakti* principle. As we will show later, the proper study of spirituality addresses this Centre of Consciousness or central core.

Now modern physics tells us that matter, including the physical body, is also an energy field (Capra, 1991; Talbot, 1981; Zukov, 1979). Physics says that we are mostly space in which there are vibrating, standing energy, "light" or matter waves which our senses present to us as an illusory solid body. Yoga says it this way:

> "Viewing the centres, (in other words the Chakras) in deep meditation, and ascending his consciousness through them in the various stages of *samadhi* or deep meditation, the Yogi has solved the mystery of the body. He knows it as a manipulatable form of light vibrations."
> Yogananda, 1995

So both East and West seem to reach the same conclusion: the one through science - mathematical physics; the other through personal realization in deep meditation. Personality in this system is everything except that central core of consciousness, which is of the fundamental nature of spirit or divinity - *sat, cit, ananda*: existence, consciousness, and bliss.

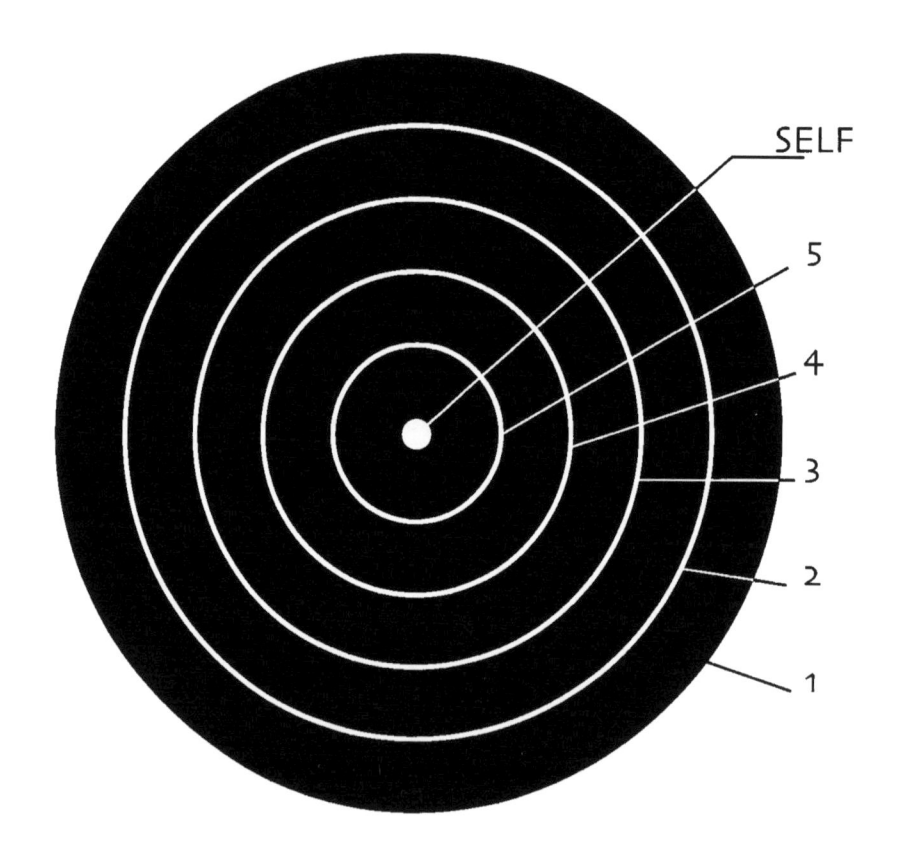

Personality Sheath | Body | States of Consciousness

Dual or Subject-Object Consciousness

	Personality Sheath	Body		States of Consciousness
1.	Annamayakosh Mental Sheath	Physical	Physical	Waking
2.	Pranamayakosha Energy Sheath	Vitality		
3.	Manomayakosha Mental Sheath	Mind	Subtle	Dreaming
4.	Vijnanamayakosha Intellectual or Intuitive Sheath Buddhi	Intelligence		
5.	Anandamayakosha	Bliss	Causal	Deep Sleep

Nondual or Consciousness-Without-an-Object

6.	SELF	Core	Turiya

"Reality is Consciousness" Aitareya Upanishad 3.3

Figure 2. The Personality According to Vedanta (Taittiriya Upanishad)

17. *The experience of physical matter is a construction of the five senses.*

Let us travel from outside, in, beginning with the physical body. Our emphasis here will be the current scientific understanding of what we would call host resistance, what some would call psychoneuroimmunology (PNI), and what others would call the healer within. For this is the core system at the physical level that is regulated by the various practices of yoga, especially meditation.

Basically the PNI paradigm extends the concept of stress to join the nervous, endocrine and immune systems into a functioning unity. The newcomer is the immune system, which is built as a stimulus-response mechanism. Like the nervous system, it recognizes the stimulus specifically and has memory built in (Jerry, 1996).

PSYCHONEUROIMMUNOLOGY
Paradigm for Host Resistance

- The immune system is a sensory organ - an extension of the nervous system.
- Both immune and nervous systems are in close communication.
- Their mutual interaction is modulated by the mind.

The hormonal and psychophysiologic (autonomic) correlates of stress are well-known. However, the PNI thesis extends the stress model to include the immune system. Many reports show that psychological factors, especially stress, can influence the immune response and, therefore, susceptibility to infectious, allergic and autoimmune diseases as well as to cancer. The missing link in trying to understand these observations is how the nervous and immune systems communicate. It had been previously thought that the immune system was autonomous in the body since one can get a full immune response in a test tube. It is now proposed that the cells of the immune system act in a sensory capacity, informing the brain about stimuli not detected by the classical sensory system, such as invading foreign pathogens or cancer cells. Both systems are in constant close communication and their mutual interaction seems to be modulated by the mind. Thus PNI is a theory about how certain aspects of the body's physiology work (2). It is not a new age therapy as some would advertise.

Some recent interesting research (Childre & Martin, 1999) in neurocardiology is shedding new light on the role that the heart may play as part of this psychosomatic network (3).

PNI is an outgrowth of Selye's general adaptation syndrome, his well-known model of stress (Selye, 1976). The concept of balance is key here. The perennial wisdom extends the concept of stress based on this central idea of adaptive balance and homeostasis.

One usually thinks of stress in terms of abnormal activation of the sympathetic side of the autonomic nervous system, leading to arousal: fight, flight and fright. But there can also be parasympathetic dominance leading to inhibition with lethargy, apathy, depression, and feelings of helplessness and hopelessness that can be seen in chronic diseases like cancer. This has been called the possum response because these individuals may react to threat with passive withdrawal, much like a possum (Nuernberger, 1979). A possum does not run away when threatened, it just rolls over and plays dead. In sutra 13 we mentioned Swami Rama's four urges which are to be controlled. The fourth is self-preservation (survival), which can be reconceptualized here as stress. The ubiquity of stress as a causative factor in ill health is now widely accepted.

At the level of mind cognitive models of the world with their component beliefs and values determine the setting of the whole system (Jerry, 1996).

Thus psychoneuroimmunology is a concept that leads to a more holistic and preventive approach to illness and wellness - a paradigm for holistic medicine.

18. *Prana (subtle energy fields) is the missing link between mind and body.*

Energy fields are the missing mind-body link. As a concept, this *pranic* or energy field/ body is also not new. There are historical references back to 5000 BCE in India, 3000 BCE in China, 500 BCE in Greece at the time of Pythagorus to a universal energy field (Brennan, 1987; Becker & Selden, 1985). It has many synonyms: *prana*, *Ch'i*, vital (energy), illiaster, magnetic fluid, odic force, aura, orgone, life field, bioplasma, etc. We will use the word prana to refer to it (Swami Rama, 1986a). From physics we are familiar with Einstein's famous equation showing the link between energy and matter. In the perennial wisdom the links are consciousness ↔ energy ↔ matter.

The human energy field is the vehicle that carries one's energy or life force. In the perennial wisdom it is primary, providing an energy matrix structure upon which cells grow. The field exists prior to the physical; the body is created by the field. Thus an imbalance or a distortion in this field eventually causes disease in that part of the physical body which it governs. Therefore, correcting distortions in the field brings about healing in the physical body.

Healing becomes learning how to correct the field by restructuring, balancing and charging it.

The events in the energy field are primary, and always precede a physical event and precipitate it. Illnesses show up in the field before they do in the physical body. They can be healed in the field before they precipitate in the physical body.

The aura is the vehicle for all psychosomatic reactions, the place where psychological processes occur. To a healer, all disease is psychosomatic. A balanced functioning of the aura is necessary to maintain health.

In the ancient wisdom, *pranayama* is the science that deals with the energy body, and the breath is the gateway. The rewards of pranayama are robust health and longevity.

But the auric field may not be the source of the event. It is a vehicle through which the creative consciousness of the spiritual core reaches the physical. In this sense one only goes back one step in the causal chain. It is said that treating the physical only treats symptoms and not the causes. The same criticism also applies to the field. One has to probe deeper to the mind, remembering that the mind itself is also a subtle energy field in yoga. We note again (sutras 15 and 16) that there are two manifestations in the universe: Consciousness (as Spirit) and energy (as *prana* or life force), each being one aspect of an underlying Unity. *Prana* expresses as a spectrum of energy fields from the subtlest (mind) through to the most gross (physical matter).

The ancient texts show that the energy field has both structure and function (Swami Rama, 1986a). It is comprised of a network of subtle *nadis* or channels through which the *prana* flows, and energy transducers called *chakras* which are arranged vertically along the central axis of the subtle body corresponding to the physical spine (Brennan, 1987; Bruyere, 1989; Pierrakos, 1975). These nadis are analogous to the acupuncture meridians (and not the physical nerves and endocrine gland or nerve plexuses as is often thought). Acupuncture also recognizes about 700 chakras where nadis cross. There are comparable concepts in Japanese systems like Judo and Shiatsu.

In Yoga 14 of these channels are important and 3 are key to spiritual practice. One is called *ida*, which runs up the left side of the spinal column but in the subtle body; one is called *pingala*, which runs up the right side, and one is called *sushumma*, that runs up the centre of the spine, but in the subtle body.

Remember that we are speaking about the subtle body, beyond the physical. These structures will not be found on an autopsy. They can be seen by psychics and by the illumined. These fields underlie therapeutic touch, Reiki, pranic healing, laying on of hands, the action of homeopathic medicines, flower essences and so on. All of these come under the science of *prana vidya*, which in Yoga is a branch of applied pranayama that includes healing techniques and intuitive diagnosis (Swami Niranjanananda, 1994).

Modern healers can "see" the energy body to various degrees and use this skill for intuitive diagnosis and energetic healing, with or without the aid of channelled guides. Some of you as readers may have this second sight already, but may not admit it for fear of censure. One of the best modern writers on the topic is Barbara Brennan. She was an atmospheric physicist cum healer who writes lucidly of her experiences in two books (Brennan 1987; 1993). She sees seven levels in the aura and beyond in great complexity with seven major chakras. She also sees other levels involving intentionality and the spiritual core. She can chart the field interactions in human relationships as well as personality types.

An altered state of consciousness is required to do this. Brennan calls it *High Sensory Perception* (HSP). Research shows that a healer's brain waves become frequency and phase synchronized with the *Schumann waves* in a process called *field coupling*. The Schumann waves are the fluctuations of the earth's magnetic field at 7.8 - 8 Hz. Healers call this "grounding into the earth". The left and right cerebral hemispheres of the healer then balance and show a similar 7.8 - 8 Hz alpha rhythm. Then later as the healing progresses, the patient's cerebral hemispheres balance with right equal to left and go alpha in synchrony with the healer as she or he links the client with the earth's magnetic field with its tremendous energy source.

19. Breath is the gateway to control of the psychoneuroimmune system and host resistance.

Now, let us introduce the role of breath into all of this; something which is a critical part of yoga and of the perennial wisdom itself (reviewed in Jerry,1996). It turns out, surprisingly, that the study of ultradian rhythms of nasal dominance, which were described in 1895 by Kayser, provide a very interesting window on the homeostatic nature of PNI function.

The nasal mucosa is erectile like the breasts and the genitals. There is an alternating cycle of nasal dominance in a 90 - 120 minute ultradian rhythm during every 24 hour period. It comes under the regulation of the autonomic nervous system where it is controlled centrally by a single oscillator, probably in the hypothalamus or perhaps in the medulla of the brain at the level of the respiratory centre. (The perennial wisdom would assign the locus of control to the pineal gland.)

The open, active, or dominant nostril shows sympathetic dominance with vasoconstriction of the nasal erectile tissues. There is an increase in mucosal gland secretion that moistens and facilitates the filtration of air by surface cilia in the lining mucous membrane with the increased air flow. The passive, closed, or non-dominant nostril shows the opposite pattern.

As the nasal cycle changes, it passes through a point of balance, where for a brief period, the air flow through the two nostrils becomes equal. This is called *sushumna* in yoga (Swami Rama, 1992; 1986a). There is an associated psychophysiological state that has been quite well characterized. Rossi (1986) thinks that it may underlie the phenomenon of spontaneous hypnosis which Milton Erickson called the "common everyday trance". He used it to facilitate his unique naturalistic approach to hypnosis which uses 90 - 120 minute sessions.

But, the plot thickens! Sperry and Gazzaniga developed the concept of hemispheric dominance based on their studies of patients who had had cerebral commissurotomies (Sperry & Gazzaniga, 1967). Initially it was thought that hemispheric dominance was fixed: people were mainly right-brained or left-brained. But subsequently it has become clear that there is a spontaneous 90 minute alteration in dominance between the left and the right cerebral hemispheres as measured during sleep on the EEG, and during wakefulness by changes in cognitive style. And yes, you guessed it! There is a direct relationship of this cerebral hemispheric activity as measured on the EEG, with the ultradian rhythm of the nasal cycle. The two are "hard-wired" together (Werntz, 1982).

It is quite possible to voluntarily change nasal dominance by forced uni-nostril breathing through the nondominant, more closed nostril. (We owe that knowledge also to yoga, as well as many other ways to change the reflex (Swami Rama, 1992; 1986a). This results in an accompanying shift in cerebral hemispheric dominance to the contralateral or opposite side. So the yogis have known that changing nasal air flow voluntarily will shift the relative activity in the highest centres of the brain, and thereby will influence the autonomic nervous system which, in turn, regulates virtually every other function of the body, including the PNI system and host resistance.

The nasal cycle is an easily measured indicator, a window, for autonomic nervous system regulation and for its integration with cerebral hemispheric activity. The whole body is thought to go through a rest/activity or parasympathetic/sympathetic oscillation, while simultaneously passing through a left body-right brain or right body-left brain shift every 90 - 120 minutes in a healthy individual. This produces dozens of ultradian rhythms at all levels of organization, from pupil size all the way up to higher cortical functions and behaviour.

Nostril dominance reflects PNI system balance. When balance is exquisite one can barely tell the difference in the dominance of the flow of the two nostrils. Their differential in flow is slight. Indeed a student can learn to consciously shift that dominance at will by mental concentration. But when the balance is not so fine the difference in flow is more striking, with one nostril almost plugged and the other open wide. When balance is seriously disturbed the ultradian rhythm becomes altered, with one nostril dominating for longer periods. When one nostril flows for a long time it is said that this predicts the onset of illness, and that deliberately shifting that dominance by one of several methods can prevent illness.

While all of this represents perhaps 50 years of Western research, it and much, much more, has been known to yoga science for probably 5000 years. It comes under a branch of yoga called *Svara Yoga* which is documented in a Tantric text called the *Shiva Svarodaya* (Swami Rama, 1986a).

20. Svara Yoga is the science of breath rhythms

Svara Yoga describes the science of the flow of these energy fields in the breath and in the nadis of the subtle body. Both words mean flow. "*Nadi*" refers to the flow of *prana shakti* (subtle energy) in the subtle body, in the *chakras* and in the 72,000 channels or *nadis*. The word "*svara*" refers to the flow of *prana shakti*, the energy fields, in the breath itself.

In terms of the breath, there are three subtle energy fields to consider. Three subtle forces or *shaktis* flow in the breath.

- *Chitta Shakti* is what is called the force of *ida*, the mental energy. This is the energy that governs thought and mind, emotion and mental activity. These are the energies that come together to create one's experience of a subjective world. In yoga the mind is a subtle energy field. There is no mind-body dichotomy in yoga. This force is associated with air flow in the dominant left nostril, associated with right cerebral hemispheric and parasympathetic dominance. It is called the *chandra*, the moon *svara*, and it gives the body a negative energy polarity.

- Then there is the opposite one, the force of *pingala* or *Prana Shakti*. This is the vital life force that governs active physical functioning. These are the forces that come together to create one's experience of the objective world. They are associated with right nostril dominant flow, as well as left hemispheric and sympathetic dominance. This is called the sun, or *surya svara* which gives a positive energy polarity to the body.

- And finally there is the *Atma Shakti*, the force of *sushumna*, the spiritual energy force. When that flows, both nostrils flow equally. The *ida* and *pingala* forces are harmonized. This is a neutral force. It influences higher dormant brain centres and the autonomic nervous system.

Sushumna is dormant in all of us unless it is awakened by yogic practice. We live entirely under the control of the other two - the subjective and objective worlds. The direct awareness of spirit is not a part of the every day experience of most of us.

These three energies also have the same 24 hour ultradian rhythm of 90 - 120 minute cycles as the breath, during which the *sushumna* force flows only for a second or two as the energies cycle between *ida* and *pingala*, between the subjective and the objective sides. It is interesting that these cycles are adjusted to the lunar fortnights (Swami Muktibodhananda Saraswati, 1983). On the bright fortnight, the first day of which is the new moon, the left nostril flows at dawn and the right at dusk. This switches like clockwork in a healthy individual every three days. During the dark fortnight, which begins with a full moon, you get the opposite pattern. It is easy to check and gives one much food for thought.

In any therapeutic program for optimizing host resistance one should include major work with the breath. At the simplest level, the breath can be used to balance consciously the neural inputs into the autonomic nervous and PNI systems. This is accomplished using diaphragmatic breathing or two-to-one breathing (with prolonged exhalation) (Swami Rama, 1992). Through innervation of the respiratory muscles, especially the diaphragm by the Hering Breuer reflex and vagus nerve, inhalation produces sympathetic input while exhalation gives parasympathetic stimulation to the system. This is most easily observed with the sinus arrhythmia associated with respiration on an electrocardiogram.

The foundation exercise for this kind of regulation is called *nadi shodhanam* or alternate nostril breathing (Swami Rama, 1992). It is useful for calming emotional disturbance, in drug dependency, in anger management, in manic depression, in resolving migraines or relieving angina from coronary spasm. The breath is the only bodily function that can be conscious or unconscious. As such it becomes a window to observe and to control host resistance and the PNI system, as well as the emotions and the mind, because these mechanisms of host resistance lie within the influence of the unconscious the mind.

21. All of the body is in the mind, but not all of the mind is in the body.

This sutra quotes a statement often made by Swami Rama. All aspirants should have a good practical working model of the human mind. Notice the word "practical". Models are important for their utility, not for their truth. When the atom used to be conceptualized as a small solar system with electrons orbiting a central nucleus like planets around the sun, the issue was not whether an atom would actually look like that if you could see it. Rather if one conceptualized it in this way one could do calculations that led to useful practical results.

It is in this spirit that we offer the model we use to conceptualize the human mind. Our model draws heavily from modern psychology, especially Neuro-Linguistic Programming (NLP), and is shown in figure 3 (p63). It matches the yogic model sufficiently closely. It can also be used to organize a wide range of therapeutic interventions that will not be covered here. But the student can use any useful model that will allow the exploration of inner space without losing one's bearings. It becomes a map to understand what is going on in the mind as the student observes. Most of us are insufficiently sensitive to our inner lives that we need a good map to interpret our inner experience as we undertake the journey to the Self.

The student will be familiar with the four-part model of the human mind commonly used in yoga. It consists of the sensory-motor mind or *manas*, and the intellect or *buddhi*, as distinct functions of the mind-stuff or mind-field called *chitta*. The latter contains the subconscious/unconscious with its residues of past action (*karma*) and experience called *samskaras*. These "seeds of karma"

THE MIND

SELF

Intuition

Cognition

Paradigms Language

BUDDHI
Higher/Inner Buddhi
Lower/Outer Buddhi

20% Deletion
Distortion
Generalization

Perception

5 Senses

IC ↔ IS → EB

IB

MANAS

5 Active Senses

Unconscious

PNI   Memory

CHITTA

Samskaras

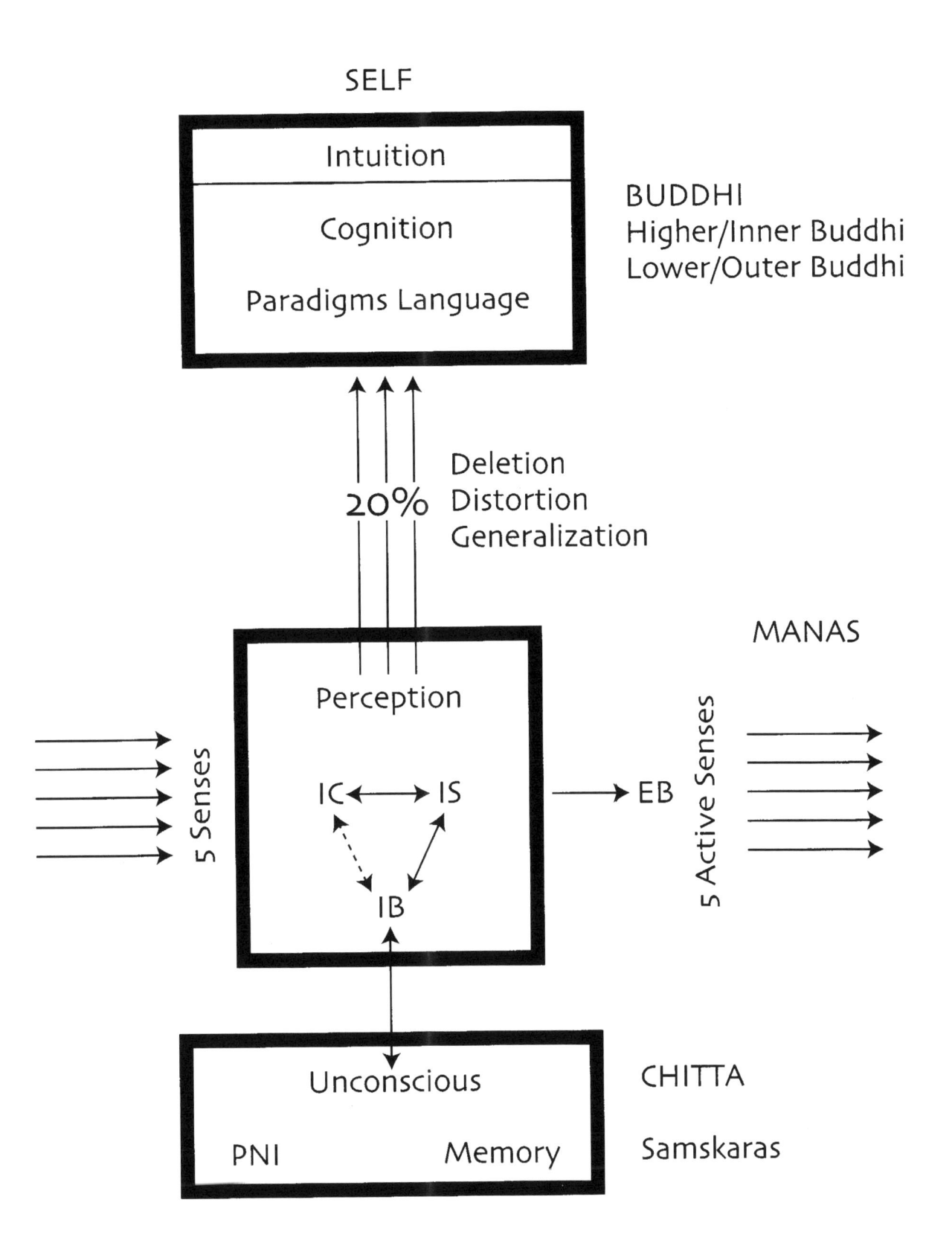

Figure 3. A Working Model of the Mind

express into behaviour when triggered by stimuli from the appropriate external context in a reactive, stimulus-response fashion. The five cognitive senses (seeing, hearing, touch, taste and smell) provide input into *manas*. The resulting output is through the five active senses (grasping, locomotion, speech, excretion and generation). The *buddhi* or intellect has an outer "face" that mediates judgment, decision and rationality. *Buddhi* also has an inner "face" of such refinement and subtlety that it can reflect spirit through intuition.

The fourth component is *ahamkara* or ego, which is not shown directly on the diagram. Ego is the principle of identification by which Consciousness identifies with various structures and functions of the mind field to create the illusion of an individualized identity, ego or "small self". When I am confronted with a horse, for example, the five cognitive senses convey imagery to *manas*. *Buddhi* identifies the imagery as a horse standing in a meadow. *Ahamkara* identifies it as "my horse", and using the five active senses I walk over to feed it a lump of sugar.

The Western model has two major levels. The first is, again, the sensory-motor mind with the same five inputs (now called representational systems) and five outputs (now identified as external behaviour (EB)). Cognition (knowing) at this level is called perception. Awareness of the sensory input can occur in various combinations of the five sensory modalities, although the visual, auditory and kinesthetic modalities are often the most dominant, with one of these being principal in any given individual. Visual and auditory images pass through the mind in rapid sequences called strategies that usually end in a kinesthetic step, which initiates an external behaviour or response. These internal sequences of imagery are called internal computations (IC). They produce internal states (IS) or feelings including but not restricted to, emotions that can initiate internal (IB) or external behaviours (EB).

Internal behaviours refer to inputs into the unconscious mind that control both memory and the psychoneuroimmune system. Autonomic responses and gestures are examples of these automatic behaviours. In this model the signs and symptoms of disease are conceptualized as internal behaviours.

Clarity and awareness of the sequences of imagery (IC) and of the internal feeling states (IS), including the emotions they elicit, as well as how behaviour flows from them, can lead to significant understanding and control of the restlessness of the mind. In this kind of analysis it is important to distinguish content from process. This model of the mind is predominantly process-oriented, and therapeutic interventions can be done to the process that are largely content free. One quickly learns that interventions designed to change process are much more effective than those aimed at changing content. Indeed, when process changes, change of content often results automatically.

We are meaning-making beings. The intellect is the second major level of mind. As cognition it constructs a model of the world in the form of belief systems about what is true, what is reality, and codes them into language. We will have much to say below about the importance of these models of the world. To do this it uses only about twenty percent of the rich material of perception by utilizing the three major processes of deletion, distortion and generalization. Deletion operates when we see only what matches our beliefs about what is true or real and we throw out contrary experience. Distortion operates frequently in science with the use of instruments like a microscope or a telescope. But it is also operative in a paranoid delusion. Generalization allows us to work all door knobs or water taps once we have mastered the use of one. But it also operates when we see all policemen as hostile after a single unhappy experience with one of them over a traffic ticket. In other words, these processes are neutral and neither good nor bad. They can have both pleasant and unpleasant outcomes depending on how they are used in a particular context. The resulting models of the world are coded in language. There are linguistic patterns that reflect and allow one to detect the operation of these three processes.

Links between these two levels of mind, perception and cognition, are very close. For example, beliefs are coded in sensory submodalities. Submodalities for vision include such things as size, shape, motion, colour, framing, etc. Auditory submodalities include volume, pitch, timbre, tonality, etc., and kinesthetic submodalities include such qualities as temperature, hardness, smoothness, wetness, etc. A strongly held belief, for example, could have images that are close, large, bright, moving, filled with sound and associated with feelings. The opposite belief might be coded as images that are distant, dim, pale, black and white, dissociated from feeling, still and quiet. Shifting key submodalities can change beliefs quickly.

There are also close links between cognition and internal states. Some of these states are a range of emotions with positive or negative qualities (the *raga* and *dvesha* of the *Yogasutras*). But others are much finer feelings and sensations. How does one know, for example, that one is secure? It is a subtle feeling. How do you know you are you when you first wake up in the morning? Indeed, how does one know that one knows? It is a kind of subtle feeling.

We have added intuition and the Self to the figure for these are generally absent from the Western models. We recommend that students spend some time becoming familiar with these or other models from personal contemplation and observation of one's own mind (e.g. Cameron-Bandler, 1985; O'Connor and Seymour, 1990).

22. *Mind continuously constructs your experience of reality through models of the world*

To consider the role of mind in this context is to discuss cognitive models and paradigms. Carl Pribram has proposed that the brain processes data consistent with what it is used to. Now what that means is that the map is not the territory. This is an old presupposition of cybernetics - that there is an irreducible difference between the world and how we experience it. We do not operate directly on the world. We create a representation of it, a map, a model. That model determines how we experience the world, and how we perceive it; our choices, our behaviour, our host resistance and physiology through the psychoneuroimmune system, and yes, even to some extent our state of health. But a map or model of the world is not the territory it represents any more than a street map is the city it represents. Both are isomorphic - have a similar structure to - the territory and thereby are useful in finding one's way around.

These models and the belief systems on which they are built are based in part on experience (compelling reference experiences in the jargon, and these can be modelled). No two people have exactly the same experiences. Therefore, each of us creates a different model of the world that we share, so that we each live in a unique reality

Now, in the twentieth century this idea originated largely from the writings of Alfred Korzybski (1980), but it has been elaborated in psychology, Neuro-Linguistic Programming (Dilts et al, 1979), and other areas, as well as in the social (Slife & Williams, 1995) and organizational sciences (Clegg et al, 1996), constructivism (Rosen & Kuehlwein, 1996; Freedman & Combs, 1996), institutional theory (Scott, 1995) and post-modernism (Clegg et al, 1996). But it is not a new concept. It really belongs to the theory of *maya* in Vedanta where it refers to the mental conditioning that has to be purified before spiritual consciousness can be experienced. We simply cannot emphasize enough the importance of this concept of models of the world for understanding the perennial wisdom.

In the postmodern view, for example, models of the world are dynamic and constantly unfolding into a life narrative (Rosen & Kuehlwein, 1996;

Freedman & Combs, 1996). Each individual develops a story about his or her life that becomes the basis of all identity. Narratives are the product of relationships, a dynamic and recursive process involving interaction with other people's perception and understanding of us (Lax, 1996). We shape our own experience of reality within a community of others. Historical, political, economic, social and cultural contexts prescribe the boundaries of our narratives. Our moment to moment evolving narrative embodies our sense of self. It reveals that self in every moment of interaction with others through the continual dance of ongoing narrative that we maintain with others.

Thus a permanent personal self or ego is merely an illusion that we cling to. It is an identification with our model of the world. It is a narrative we develop in relation to others over time that we come to identify as who we are. The personal self is a fiction.

This concept has important parallels in Eastern thought. The things we "see" are only the concepts stemming from our narrative structures, rather than what is really there. The Buddha taught that one should see things as they really are. We are to view the world realizing that how we experience it is our construction based on our desires and fears. We continually create our experience of the world, of reality, based on our beliefs. We grasp at what brings us pleasure and we push away what causes us pain. But our construction is changing, a dynamic narrative, and because nothing can be held onto or repelled forever then all of our effort leads to suffering if we get caught up in this cyclical attraction and avoidance process (called *raga* and *dvesha* in the *Yogasutras* of Patanjali (Aranya, 1981)). Indeed, in the yoga philosophy a metaphor is often used where life is considered to be a book with no beginning and no ending, the pages of which we write as our life story from day to day and moment to moment.

These models of the world or mental paradigms obey "laws". Like the psychoneuroimmune system at the molecular and physiological levels, they tend to be homeostatic; they are self-regulating and resist change. They operate mostly below the daily level of awareness, and likely influence physiology through the unconscious mind, or the right brain as some would suggest. These unconscious models can then produce behaviour which may seem irrational, or be dismissed as emotional or reactive. Rather, if one knew the underlying model with its beliefs and values, in fact the behaviour would be quite rational. If we take an example, part of the business of mind-body medicine is modelling dysfunctional belief systems in disease so that they can be changed to generate a secondary effect in the physiology of host resistance. More effective psychological coping leads to a beneficial rebalancing of host resistance and the psychoneuroimmune system.

Paradigms can be modelled in terms of both content and structure. Their content is made up operationally of cause-effects and criteria, the latter referring to the values, beliefs, and expectations we use to codify, judge and make meaning out of our everyday experience. As discussed above these internal models of the world represent a secondary level of experience, often coded in language, and produced by the intellectual faculties through distortion, deletion and generalization, in linguistic terms, of primary sensory experience as represented by mental imagery linked to affect and stored in the unconscious mind (Grinder & Bandler, 1975; 1976). Strong beliefs form from life's compelling reference experiences linked to strong affect or emotion.

Primary data in the form of images in memory and their associated affect can be accessed (and altered) by various techniques, for example hypnosis (Rossi & Cheek, 1988), reframing (Bandler and Grinder, 1982; Cameron-Bandler, 1985), altering the submodalities of the imagery (Bandler, 1985), changing the arrangement of the structure of that internal subjective experience of space, time and neurology (James & Woodsmall, 1988), or through the use of meridian therapies from the new energy psychology (Gallo, 1999). A knowledge of some of these methods can be helpful to the spiritual aspirant or *sadhaka* in mitigating some of the unpleasantness of repressed material as it is released from the unconscious mind during the purification of intense *sadhana* or spiritual practice. Purification need not entail emotional pain and suffering as some would have you believe. Indeed wallowing in the emotion as suppressed material surfaces can have the opposite effect of strengthening the emotional charge and the attachment.

23. *Manifested reality is holographic. There is both a cosmic and an individual person. The microcosm reflects the macrocosm.*

In his book, *Global Mind Change*, Willis Harmon (1988) describes three basic metaphysics which have been used during the history of human evolution (Slife & Williams, 1995). M-1 or Materialistic Monism refers to matter giving rise to mind, to mind out of matter. Matter-energy is the basic stuff of the universe and consciousness is a product of it (of the brain). This world view underlies most of our current western cultural heritage. It supports the mechanistic science of the West, including modern molecular medicine. M-2 or Dualism postulates both matter and mind. There are two fundamentally different basic "stuffs" in the universe: matter-energy which is the subject of science, and mind-spirit which is studied by the psychic and the mystic. The two are forever separate. Finally, M-3 or Transcendental Monism involves mind giving rise to matter - matter out of mind. In this view the ultimate stuff in the universe is consciousness. Mind/consciousness is primary, and matter-energy comes out of mind like a dream. One contacts the reality behind the phenomenal world by the intuition and not by the physical senses.

The M-3 metaphysics is similar to Tantra which views the universe as consciousness (*Shiva*) enrobed in energy (*Shakti*). It also reminds one of the Vedantic *maya*, where the true Self is pure consciousness - ever pure, ever wise, ever free: *sat, chit, ananda*, which is obscured by the coverings of *maya*. This metaphysics is closer to David Bohm's interpretation of quantum physics with implicate and explicate realities (Bohm, 1983; Bohm & Peat, 1987). But Harmon confuses mind with spirit. In the *Yogasutras* mind is presented as a very refined energy field (Aranya, 1981). Its upper reaches are so refined (the higher Buddhi) that it can reflect the Self, the *Atman*, the *Purusha*, pure consciousness, Spirit. So one conceives of an energy spectrum ranging from matter ("frozen light") through to mind. In this conception there is no mind-body problem or dichotomy. Rather the discontinuity is between spirit or consciousness and energy (4).

This is a dynamic process. From moment to moment one is an unfolding self. Life is a rhythmic pulse between manifestation and the Centre of Consciousness - that great void and plenum within the core of one's being, which is the essence of the unfolding spiritual awareness. This expansion and contraction takes place every moment: a multifold expansion/stasis and then contraction/stasis pulse. Fast pulses and slow pulses. David Bohm describes it as movement between the implicate and explicate realities - a dynamic process he refers to as the holomovement. Tantra describes it as the out-winking and the in-winking of the *shakti*. Indian philosophy uses the metaphor of the breath, or of the circle with a central point, with contraction and expansion between the centre and the periphery. The centre is everywhere (the Centre of Consciousness is an unchanging, given experience no matter where you are in space and time), and the circumference is nowhere (the infinite expansion of consciousness). To exist is a dynamic and creative process from that spiritual core. In this sense you create your experience of your world around you as well as your state of health through an expansion/stasis and communication with the universe around you, followed by a contraction/stasis and communion with your interior individuality. You are an unfolding self, and your state of health unfolds moment by moment as an individual and dynamic state.

24. *The Centre of Consciousness from which consciousness flows in various degrees and grades, lies at the core of the personality.*

What does the perennial wisdom say about consciousness? Referring back again to figure 2, which we have dubbed the "Vedantic target" as a symbolic map of the personality, we are now concerned with what is labelled as Self at the centre. Our journey to now has been through body, energy system and mind to this central point. In this model manifested reality, the universe, is consciousness (*shiva* or *purusha*) enrobed in layers of energy (*shakti, maya, prakriti*). These interpenetrating layers of energy create a vibrational spectrum reaching from mind to matter (physical body). The layers of this vibrational spectrum are called *koshas* (energy sheaths), which collectively make up what is called the personality. Consciousness pervades the personality like space pervades and holds the contents of a room.

The model works at both cosmic and individual levels. There is a cosmic person making up the *macrocosm* of which the personality (or embodiment) is the cosmos, and an individual person or *microcosm*. The model is holographic in that all of the universe is enfolded in both levels - implicit in the Hermetic phrase, "As above, so below." The experience of physical matter is a construction of the five senses. It might be considered as "frozen energy" in the form of standing waves. Such a model is consistent with the ideas of modern physics.

For the study of consciousness, the issue focuses on what is the Self at the centre of the target. The answer in Vedanta is pure Consciousness. Spirit and Consciousness are the same. The ultimate reality is Consciousness. Thus a consideration of Consciousness means a consideration of spirituality and vice versa (5).

In dealing with the phenomenal world the philosophy looks at two levels of knowledge or *vidya* that are to be attained. *Apara vidya* is the lower knowledge. It is the knowledge of the created world and phenomenal experience with which we are all familiar. It has a causal order in time and space, and it also carries moral consequence through the doctrine of *karma* (causality). It involves a process of knower, the object of knowledge and the instrument of knowledge that occurs with subject-object consciousness or consciousness-with-an-object. In contrast, there is *para vidya* or the higher knowledge. This is direct knowledge of Reality. It is not the effect or cause of anything and lies beyond either karmic consequence or transmigratory existence which is called *samsara*. It is of the nature of Consciousness-without-an-object, the awareness of the identity of the knowing subject with Reality.

25. *The Atman or Self at the core is pure Consciousness. The ultimate reality is Consciousness or Spirit.*

What has Advaita Vedanta to say about Consciousness? This philosophy is considered to be one of the broadest and most comprehensive theories of consciousness in any philosophical tradition east or west (6). It is built on a doctrine of radical discontinuity between the absolute and phenomenal states of consciousness. There is an absolute or pure universal consciousness called *cit*, or *sakshi caitanya*. There is also a phenomenal or modified consciousness called *citta* or *vrtti caitanya*. In other words consciousness is awareness, intelligence or knowledge (in the sense of knowing) that may be free or bound. The higher order consciousness is the underlying unifying intelligent ground of all phenomenal states of consciousness. "Reality is consciousness" (Aitareya Upanishad 3.3). This higher order consciousness, called *sutratma*, is likened to a thread that courses through and holds together a collection of pearls.

Phenomenal consciousness is arranged in a hierarchical nature in which the phenomena are ordered according to their respective degrees of subtlety or purity and intelligence. They become a hierarchy of psychological states. These are described in the Mandukya Upanishad (Swami Nikhilananda, 1987) as the four quarters of Self (*Atman*) or pure Consciousness. They are the waking, dream and deep sleep states with which we are all familiar and a "fourth" (*turiya*) that is the true Consciousness, the Witness that underlies the other three and remains unaffected as It moves through them. The other three states are in order of subtlety in terms of their objects of experience. They are ordered with increasing purification and intensification of consciousness. Each state demonstrates its function as the enjoyer.

In this system value means the ability to discriminate the real from the non-real, phenomenal from absolute consciousness. It is the ability to go beyond conceptual knowledge about Reality to actual realization of Reality and liberation itself. This is the path of Jnana Yoga which is a progressive de-superimposition of Self from non-Self. This ultimate Consciousness or Reality is an unalterably Self-shining, Self -revealing, pure Consciousness. The process is not an increasing realization of Consciousness, but rather the process is a decrease in the veiling power of ignorance, decreasing levels of ignorance, decreasing degrees of obscuration of this eternally Self-luminous and pure Consciousness. This becomes the ultimate goal of life. It also implies that people will differ in levels of awareness or consciousness depending on their degree of development. One's job is to climb the ladder to a higher degree of realization of one's potential.

This hierarchy of psychological states has a correspondence to the five sheaths or *koshas* as described in the Taittiriya Upanishad (Swami Nikhilananda, 1977a) and diagrammed in figure 2 above. With waking consciousness one is identified with the physical or gross body which is the *annamayakosha* or gross body (*sthula-sharira*). Then there is a subtle body (*suksma-sharira*) which is identification with the dream state. It contains three sheaths; vitality (*pranamayakosha*), mind (*manomayakosha*) and intelligence or understanding (*vijnanamayakosha*). At the most subtle level is the *karana-sharira* or causal body. Identification with it is deep sleep and represents the most subtle and pure sheath of bliss, the *anandamayakosha*. In this sense causal means the experience of a blank, of a pure ignorance, an undifferentiated veiling quality of the underlying pure Consciousness which is the cause of the previous sheaths and limits association with them. These levels range from the least real or gross to the more real or subtle levels.

26. *The scientific study of spirituality is the scientific study of Consciousness.*

This brief consideration of consciousness in sutra 25 uncovers some major sources of confusion to our understanding of spirituality in Western science.
- The lack of a clear definition of spirituality. One cannot use the scientific method to study something that is not clearly defined.
- A confusion among the definitions, roles and functions of brain, emotions, mind, consciousness and spirit.
- Through lack of appreciation of the existence and role of the *pranamaya kosha* within the human personality, there is a confusion of subtle prana with spirit and also with physical electromagnetic fields, as well as a confusion of pranic forms of healing ("energy" or "vibrational" medicine) with spiritual healing. From an Eastern perspective of Spirit as Absolute Consciousness, Spirit, the Self, is in no need of healing! Indeed, Self-Recognition may be considered the ultimate healing as the transcendence of the ultimate disease - *samsara* or cyclic phenomenal existence.
- There is a confusion of science with technology. Science is simply a systematic way of learning from experience - of gaining valid knowledge through valid experimental method and analysis. The technology is only the instrument for this process.

But nowhere does the gulf between science and spirituality seem greater than in the reductionistic and materialistic assumptions that underlie modern Western science - except perhaps the recent trend to postmodern subjectivism. Some advocates of this child of modern philosophy, operating in science through qualitative research methods, promote an undisguised attack on experimental positivistic science (Koertge, 1998; Sokal and Bricmont, 1998). They espouse the relativity and subjectivity of truth - the notion that "it's true because I (or the majority) believe or feel it". This attitude is beginning to pervade modern culture, politics, environmentalism and social science.

27. *Yoga is the science of spirituality.*

In sutra 23 we referred to Willis Harmon's description of three forms of metaphysics that underlie models of the nature of mind. This concept can be modified to apply to our consideration of consciousness as follows:

- M-1 Metaphysics is materialistic monism.
  Consciousness is derived out of matter or energy.
- M-2 Metaphysics is dualism.
  Consciousness plus matter/energy both exist.
- M-3 Metaphysics is transcendental monism.
  Matter/energy are derived out of Consciousness.

Clearly the Western scientific approach is based in M-1 metaphysics, while the Eastern philosophies which are based on the revelations of Recognition by awakened sages, are based on M-3 metaphysics. The two approaches are polar opposites!

In the West, what defines a body of knowledge as scientific or as an empiric science? According to Merrell-Wolff (1994, p246) there are only two necessary conditions: 1. "The interpretive theory must be a logical and self-consistent whole from which deductive inferences can be drawn", and 2. "The theory ... [should] ... suggest an empirically possible experiment or observation that can confirm or fail to confirm the inference." The latter pragmatic condition distinguishes modern science from the purely subjective rationalism of the scholastics and of Aristotle. It is the key to the modern control of nature and to the western development of technology. An organized collection of observed facts that satisfies these two conditions is an empiric science in the current sense of the word.

But Merrell-Wolff (1994, p108) is even stronger in his assertion that because science as practised in the West (and language through which it is expressed), can only deal with the manifested universe, subject-object consciousness, the universe of the senses, perception and cognition, it cannot grasp the Transcendent. Some linguistic ideas about the "Truth" can emerge but the "Thing-in-itself" is never realized any more than a blind person can know the universe of sight no matter how much intellectual effort is expended. The secret remains a secret no matter how openly it is debated. "God [Spirituality], Consciousness is either Known directly through Identity, or He is not known at all." (Merrell-Wolff, 1994, p65). This "Knowledge through Identity" or direct apperception of Truth refers to the awakened faculty of intuition in yoga.

But there is a further criterion that modern science raises as a condition of its advance. Interpretation of experimental data should be consistent with the current scientific point of view. "So long as it is not 'necessary' to change, it is necessary 'not' to change." (Merrell-Wolff, 1994, p247). This has profound implications for conservatism and for the difficulty of achieving paradigm shifts in science. This conservativism applies also to medical science and especially medical practice. Indeed, the medical profession is among the most conservative of forces in modern society. And well it should be for very few of the "advances" in the latest medical journals ever survive the test of time to become established parts of the standard medical armamentarium.

But the new world view, the paradigm shift that liberates, soon becomes the paradigm that binds. Since it is a construction of the ego the new paradigm binds with even stronger chains than the old one it replaced. The result is *"paradigm blindness"*. It becomes a kind of projection leading to a theory of everything. To the quantum physicists, everything reduces down to collapsing wave functions under the conscious act of measurement. Or everything from mind to emotions to consciousness, spirit and even soul reduces to peptides of the psychosomatic network (Pert,1997) or to molecular information transduction (Rossi, 1993). To the cognitivists all can be explained by an enactive approach to cognition that brings forth a world from a history of structural coupling within a network of multiple levels of interconnected, sensory-motor sub-networks (Varela et al 1991, p206.).

But this third condition of congruence with established theory is "no real part of science as science and may not be properly invoked to discredit the 'truth' of any interpretive construction." (Merrell-Wolff, 1994, p247.). Paradigms and technology mutually interact in a dynamic way in advancing the leading edge of research. Paradigms create as well as constrain the possible questions that can be asked, while methodology limits further what can be practically investigated as feasible. But necessity as the mother of invention continually advances technological innovation and what is feasible to investigate

- hence the expanding edge of research inquiry.

Is all lost then? Can there be no science of spirituality by definition? On the contrary, the study of spirituality is actually the study of consciousness. One needs to incorporate the perennial wisdom, which does offer a pragmatic and experimental science of spirituality. It has many names and forms but at its core it is the science of yoga - a term that is still greatly misunderstood. if not mistrusted in the West. Here its major manifestation is physical postures. But it is also used in holistic health and as a complementary therapy. North American culture has modified and glamorized it until it no longer resembles its original form as a science of spirituality.

As a therapeutic modality, yoga in the West is known as an ancient system of relaxation and rejuvenation that originated in India about 6000 years ago. Its focus in the West is still hatha yoga. Postures, breath, relaxation and meditation are used to optimize physical and emotional health. The postures strengthen and tone the body and internal organs, while the exercises for breath control energize the body and calm the mind. Relaxation and meditation are used for stress relief and to clarify thinking. The practitioner learns respect for the body and personality, and the importance of being present in each moment with awareness.

Since the early 1970's, there have been over one thousand good research studies of meditation and yoga published in the medical and scientific literature. It is still little appreciated that most of the methods used for modern stress management come from yoga. The medical literature suggests that in up to 80% of all illnesses stress plays a role. Yoga is now widely used as a simple and effective tool for stress management. In 1984 the National Institutes of Health recommended meditation over prescription drugs as the first treatment for mild hypertension. The research on meditation and yoga points to their effectiveness in alleviating stress and anxiety, in reducing blood pressure and heart rate, in improving memory and intelligence, alleviating pain and improving motor skills. The research documents relief from addictions, a heightening of visual and auditory perceptions, and enhancement of metabolic and respiratory function (source, International Association of Yoga Therapists - IAYT).

But these considerable therapeutic benefits of yoga are merely byproducts of its primary purpose as a science of spirituality, of Self-Realization. Like any science its methods are precise. And here we must take issue with a disturbing trend in western research to specify poorly or even to corrupt or alter these precise methods, especially with meditation. The enormous sophistication of a western clinical trial cannot make up for a poorly defined or incorrectly used intervention. The result will still be uninterpretable.

The approach of yoga differs from that of positivistic science but its results are no less robust. In yoga the practitioner is the researcher, the object of the research, and the instrument of the research. There is no room here for the disinterested and objective observer of the positivistic scenario. Just as in quantum theory, the researcher in yoga is a full participant in the research process and, moreover, is transformed as a result. The process is very precise and the outcomes, the signposts along the way, mark its progress. The whole endeavour is more like the training of an Olympic athlete, a skilled surgeon, a mathematician, a concert pianist or an artist. "Yoga is skill in action" (Bhagavad Gita II.50). One thinks nothing of spending ten to twenty years of intense concentrated effort to achieve the heights of these worldly endeavours. Why would one think that a similar effort would not be required to achieve superconsciousness? The choice of effort boils down to one of values, of mission, of what is the most important use of the resources of an individual life.

The goal will require the union of philosophy, science, and spirituality. The term mysticism (to represent experiential spirituality), but not religion as a temporal force in society, would better describe the component to be bridged. The link between science and philosophy is currently the strongest. For although modern scientific training rarely seems to address its philosophical underpinnings, the truly great among scientists are also philosophers, especially in physics. Also the bridging between philosophy and spirituality is being forged from idealism and monism as exemplified in Harman's M-3 metaphysics. But the chasm between science and spirituality remains deep. Some attempts at bridging from science can be seen in the new scientific attempts to study subtle energies, spirituality, consciousness and meditation. At least we are talking about it!

II THE EXPERIENCE

Mystical Experience of the Centre of Consciousness

28. We are citizens of two worlds.

Swami Rama would often say that we live in two worlds. For most of us the real world is the external or outer world that we experience through our five senses. We have only the vaguest impression of an inner life in the form of emotions, thoughts, dreaming or day-dreaming. Subjective experience is commonly dismissed as unreal, and is looked upon with contempt by western material science. Even western psychology, as a science of mind, still discounts subjectivity in favour of the study of objective behaviour.

But in yoga subjective reality is recognized as being as important as objective reality. Indeed, the inner world is considered to be more real because it is the cause of external manifestation. The subtle gives rise to the gross. It is within the inner world that the Centre of Consciousness arises. Even for those who are well acquainted with the inner world, the whisperings of the Centre of Consciousness are subtler still. The inner world is much more rich, complex and variegated than the outer world. The aspirant will need to be very familiar with the landscape of the inner world before the whisperings of the Centre of Consciousness can be appreciated. The student will have one foot planted securely in each of these worlds. He or she should be comfortable in either world and be able to move between the two with ease. The distinction between the phenomena in each of these worlds should be quite clear and not confused. There should be a balance in the two experiences.

What manifests in the outer world originates causally from the inner. Swami Rama would often advise a student to take a particular course of action. The puzzled student could not understand why this advice had been given, seemingly out of nowhere, and would fail to follow through. About six months later the student would ask Swamiji if the advice could now be followed, since trouble had arrived. But Swamiji would say it was now too late to act. He used to say that events had their subtle equivalents in the inner world about six months prior to external manifestation.

People still search for God outside of themselves. Or they try to fulfill the emptiness within with a substitute like wealth, achievements, occupation or relationships. One must look within to find the divine core that lies at the centre of every personality. Initially this Centre is recognized as an object in subject-object consciousness, since the small self operates in this mode. Much later that Presence will fill not only the inner world, but all of manifestation with Its effulgence.

29. *The awakening of the Centre of Consciousness is a qualitatively new and unique experience in the inner world.*

With the awakening of the Centre of Consciousness the student is presented with a new experience that is qualitatively unique. The inner world is a complex kaleidoscope of many inputs, a rich landscape of many events and objects.

Depending on the level of awareness individuals experience various subgroups of this mental content with an expanding ability to discriminate finer and finer experiences. These potential experiences range from internal imagery through feelings, concepts, language and kinesthetics to mention but a few. But the awakening of the Centre of Consciousness is something qualitatively new and entirely different from anything experienced before.

If the experiences consist in any way of the usual mental contents, no matter how compelling, then this is not the Centre of Consciousness. This is not an expansion of awareness to include more of the same thing or a refined appreciation of the same kind of mental contents. Rather it is a discontinuous leap of the awareness to a transpersonal realm, a Presence that is experienced qualitatively as something entirely new.

It is because of this, and the lack of any referents in ordinary language, that it becomes so difficult to describe or discuss this new experience, especially among those for whom it is not yet recognized. For this reason, it is truly a secret which when revealed remains a secret. But more than that, the experience is not the simple addition of a new object to the inner world. It is a rather that the space of the inner world, the *cidakasha* itself becomes alive. Until now the experience of the inner world was only the objects that it contains. Now it is as though one can experience the very space of consciousness itself which is the container of the ordinary objects of the inner world. Hence the use in description in the texts of terms like "sky, space, void," etc.. This subtlety adds to the difficulty of its description since it cannot be referred to simply as another new object in inner space.

But first one needs a stable peace and silence in the mind, otherwise experiences will not be permanent. True consciousness can only manifest in the silent mind.

30. *It is possible to experience Spirit and not to recognize It.*

If you could experience Spirit right now, would you recognize It? It is possible to have that experience of Divinity and not recognize it. Even some great mystics have not recognized the experience at first and needed the guidance of their preceptors to understand what was happening.

Swami Rama (1999b) tells how after much insistence his master finally agreed to show him God. "I promise to show you God tomorrow morning." Swamiji spent a restless night in excited anticipation. The next morning he arose early and approached his master in excitement to remind him of his promise.

After some discussion his master leaned toward the expectant Swamiji and asked him what kind of a God he would like to see. Swamiji asked to see the God from the scriptures who is full of peace, happiness and bliss. His master replied, "But that is within you! You are searching for it outside of yourself in mundane life. You are searching for God in the wrong place!"

Based on our upbringing, our family, social and religious influences, most of us have some kind of preconception of what God is if we do believe in such a being. This preconception can prevent us from appreciating the actual experience.

> "All developed mental men, those who get beyond the average, have in one way or other, or at least at certain times and for certain purposes, to separate the two parts of the mind, the active part, which is a factory of thoughts and the quiet masterful part which is at once a Witness and a Will, observing them, judging, rejecting, eliminating, accepting, ordering corrections and changes, the Master in the House of Mind."
> Sri Aurobindo, 1972, p83

31. The initial experience of the Centre of Consciousness can be disturbing.

The unexpected recognition of something qualitatively new in the mind, however subtle, can be initially quite disconcerting. One may have a sense when one is alone of being watched, that there may be an intruder in the room. One can experience episodes of anxiety leading even to panic. It is important that the student seek advice from the preceptor as this experience unfolds. The master will be very helpful in assisting the student to identify what is happening, and to guide the student so that he or she does not confuse the experience with other mental content such as material emerging from the unconscious mind.

We had the opportunity to ask our preceptor, Swami Rama, what this Presence was in the mind. With no hesitation he quietly replied, "It is the Lord" as though this were the most ordinary thing in the world! Little did we realize at the time the future import of his seemingly casual observation. The text, Light on the Path, also makes reference to this issue.

> "The abyss of nothingness has to be faced ... The utter silence ... comes as a more appalling horror then even the formless emptiness of space. Our only mental conception of blank space is, ... when it reduced to its barest element of thought, that of black darkness. This is a great physical terror to most persons, and when regarded as an eternal and unchangeable fact, must mean to the mind the idea of annihilation rather than anything else.
> Collins, 1976, pp55-56

32. The universe of manifestation is like one's own dream-creation, like an image reflected in a mirror.

And what of the universe of manifestation? Some liken it to a dream:

> "In this infinite consciousness it is a mere fantasy that appears to be the created universe. ... It is like one's own dream-creation. ... Because the dreamer is a conscious being, the dream-objects appear to have an intelligence and a mind of their own; even so, this non-creation known as the universe seems to possess independent existence and intelligence as if it had been created. There is no creation as such : the one Brahman [Consciousness] exists as Brahman. Whatever notion [belief, idea, thought] arises in this Brahman is experienced in this Brahman as if it were a [real] object of experience."
> Yoga Vasishtha VI.2:57

Others use the analogy of the Consciousness as a mirror:

> "Just as an object is reflected in a mirror, so does this world appear in Brahman [Consciousness]. Though the reflection seems to be in the mirror, it is not [really] there: even so, though the world appears to be, it is not [really] there."
> Yoga Vasishtha VI.2:99

> "...this consciousness is the only existence. ...the universe has...originated only as an image on the surface of the mirror of the Absolute. .... Creation is like a magician's trick, and is a city born of divine imagination. ...Mirrors are insentient and are not self-contained. Whereas, consciousness is always pure and self-contained; it does not require an external object to create the image. ...The universe is nothing but an image on our consciousness. Consciousness shines notwithstanding the formation of images on it. ...Just as the images in a mirror are not apart from the mirror, so also the creations of consciousness are not apart from it. ...Note how day-dreams and hallucinations are clearly pictured in the mind even in the absence of any reality behind them. ...When such imagination is deep, it takes shape as creation; consciousness is pure and unblemished in the absence of imagination. ...So the world is nothing but an image drawn on the screen of consciousness; it differs from a mental picture in its long duration; that is again due to the strength of will producing the phenomenon. The universe appears practical, material and perfect because the will determining its creation is perfect and independent; whereas the human conceptions are more or less transitory according to the strength or weakness of the will behind them."
> Tripura Rahasya, XI:31-69.

Because of the changing images in a mirror, the reflecting surface is invisible. An animal or a child initially sees the images as real. In a metaphorical sense, to realize, to directly experience the primary reality of the reflecting "surface" of the mirror (or consciousness) itself apart from the images reflected in it is to know transcendent consciousness.

33. *It is a secret that once revealed remains a secret.*

Swami Rama was once asked to sit as an examiner to a PhD student at a leading University in South India. The student was reputed to be brilliant, and to have produced a philosophical masterpiece for his thesis. Passing the oral defence and getting his degree would be a mere formality.

When all were assembled for the debate, Swamiji was formally introduced and then the chairman gave the signal to begin. The other examiners in turn asked a series of very difficult questions. The candidate answered each brilliantly. Then came Swamiji's turn.
"How are you, son?" he asked. "This is an elegant piece of work."
"Yes, Sir." the candidate said proudly.
"Tell me, son, what are your spiritual practices?" asked Swamiji.
"Practices? I don't do any practices!" declared the candidate loudly, referring to fools like sadhus with contempt.
The room became silent. Gently and kindly Swamiji said to the candidate, "Son, it is only through direct experience that the One Truth can be known."
He then turned to the other examiners and tossing the heavy thesis on the table, said, "All of this is useless speculation. I fail the candidate." Then he stood up and walked out of the room.

The experience of the transcendent, of THAT, is ineffable. All of the texts use metaphors or indirect means to refer to IT. Language as the medium of thought cannot encompass the transcendent. It can be known only by direct experience. Then all language and description become irrelevant. Until then IT remains a secret that even though revealed still remains a secret. Since the Centre of Consciousness is an expression of THAT, Its experience is similarly ineffable.

34. *The Sages describe IT as THAT. There is no substitute for direct Realization.*

How does one speak of such an ineffable realization, of a secret that once revealed remains a secret, to the unrealized? The sages use words like "That", or "IT".

> "...as directly realized IT is a Consciousness so utterly different from anything that can be conceived by the relative consciousness that only negations can be predicated of IT. ....There is no substitute for the Direct Realization."
>
> Merrell-Wolff, 1994, p401.

35. The Centre of Consciousness is Consciousness-Without-an-Object.

Merrell-Wolff (1994) uses the phrase Consciousness-Without-an-Object to describe his experience of the transcendent. In that experience the observer, the instrument of observation, and the observed all collapse into a unity - an expanded state of the purest Being. This tripartite experience is characteristic of subject-object consciousness in which the ego and ordinary mind normally exist. It is characteristic of the universe of time, space and causation, to which the mental field also belongs.

But the Centre of Consciousness lies beyond time space and causation in the eternal NOW. To become aware of it, however dimly at this stage, means that one "stands" in awareness with one "foot" in the mind and one "foot" beyond the mind, so to speak. One takes a stance at the border between the personal and transpersonal. For at this stage on the Path the revelation of the Self is only partial. It has only just begun like the rising of the sun at the break of dawn. Much later, that revelation will become full like the brilliance of the sun at noon.

36. The Centre of Consciousness is a still, but effulgent, Conscious Presence, Silence or "Thatness". It is a Void or Emptiness that paradoxically is also a Plenum or Fullness. It pervades all of inner space and holds all manifestation, all inner mental content within Itself like space pervades and holds the contents of a room, and yet is unaffected by them.

Let us sample the record of experience of those who have realized this consciousness. If we look at the second chapter of the Bhagavad Gita there is a well known discussion of the immortality of the Self and the body as a garment to be cast off.

> "As one removes old garments and puts on new ones,
> so does the master of the body take off the worn
> flesh to wear the new one."
>
> Bhagavad Gita II.22

The infinite existence of the Spiritual Being that is our essential nature is stressed:

> "Know that as indestructible by which all this
> tangible world is permeated.
> No one has the power to bring to destruction this
> unalterable entity."
> Bhagavad Gita II.17

> "He is never born nor does He die, nor having been,
> does He ever again cease to be.
> Unborn, eternal, perennial, this ancient One is not
> killed when the body is killed."
> Bhagavad Gita II.20

> "Weapons do not cleave Him, fire does not burn Him,
> the waters do not wet him, nor does the wind dry him.
> He is uncleavable, unburnable, cannot be made wet,
> nor can He be made dry;
> The eternal, all permeating, absolute, and unmoving;
> He is the ancient One.
> He is unmanifest, is not the subject of thought and
> is said to be incorruptable;
> Therefore, knowing Him, it does not behoove you to
> grieve after anyone."
> Bhagavad Gita II.23-25.

Says the sage, Vasishtha, to Rama, "I am the pure, space-like consciousness devoid of objective experience and beyond all mental activity or thought. I am the pure and infinite consciousness. Even so are you. The whole world is that, too. Everything is the pure, indivisible consciousness." (Yoga Vasishtha VI.2:29)

The English poet Alfred Lord Tennyson has written of his own realization which occurred to him in association with repeating his name as a mantra (quoted in James, 1902/1929, p 374).

> "I have never had any revelations through anesthetics, but a kind of waking
> trance — this for lack of a better word – I have frequently had, quite up from
> boyhood, when I have been all alone. This has come upon me through
> repeating my own name to myself silently, till all at once, as it were out of
> the intensity of the consciousness of individuality, individuality itself seemed
> to dissolve and fade away into boundless being and this not a confused state
> but the clearest, the surest of the surest, utterly beyond words – were it death
> was an almost laughable impossibility – the loss of personality (if so it were)
> seeming no extinction, but the only true life. I am ashamed of my
> description Have I not said the state is utterly beyond words?"

But such awakenings appear even today. Here is a description by an individual living in Vancouver in Canada, of an experience of The One.

> "The most sincere attempt to describe what happened as I began to Ascend again does not do justice to this sacred and joyous experience. The Attitudes seemed like the softest of whispers of wind as they floated across the ocean of quietude. Instead of making ripples as a stone would do when touching the surface of the water, the Attitudes left no mark of their own as they sank into this stillness and became One with it. I allowed myself to merge with the stillness and It took me into Itself as The One fed my soul with deep and abiding Peace beyond understanding and reasoning. From this quiet ocean of Peace arose the most certain of all knowledge, yet it felt like the finest and most gentle of mists on a lake when the awakening morning sun rays kiss its surface. It told me that God is I and I am God; that indeed, I Am That. I continued to Ascend and drink of this cup of Truth which has eluded me for so long.
>
> All of Creation was contained in this. There was no doubt in my mind that I was experiencing my Self. I finally understood what the teachers desire to convey with the statement that the deepest rest is gained while Ascending. The rest was filled with total awareness of All There Is. It was many hours before I dropped off to a peaceful sleep.
>
> I still feel this Oneness. Although my experience of It has varying levels of depth since that night, my memory of It All serves me and urges me to choose over and over again. My thoughts are softer. My trust is deepening. My days are more peaceful. I forgive myself. I know that God takes care of all my needs and wants. I feel gentleness behind my eyes as I look out at the world around me. I am willing to extend love."
>
> MaLa Sahan, Vancouver, Canada, 1999.

37. Space is Self and Self is Space. In inner space the wise find the Intelligence of pure Consciousness, and ultimate Truth in the effulgent Void.

It is spoken of metaphorically. One of the commonest metaphors is that of space or sky. We would describe the experience as a still, effulgent, Conscious Presence or "Thatness", at once experienced both as a void or emptiness and also as a plenum or fullness, which holds manifestation within itself like space pervades and holds the contents of a room and yet is unaffected by them. We use the word "Presence."

> "Is there a difference between pure consciousness and utter void? ...I am the pure space of consciousness. ...It is as if void is the ultimate truth!"
> (Yoga Vasishtha VI.2:29)

> "Absolute Consciousness and space resemble each other in being perfect, infinite, subtle, pure, unbounded, formless, imminent in all, yet undefiled within and without. ...In fact, the conscious Self is space. ...Space is Self; and Self is space. ...The wise ... find in space the Self, the Abstract Intelligence."
> (Tripura Rahasya, XVIII:72-79).

To conclude this attempt at an experiential portrayal of the realization of Consciousness, let us turn to the writings of a contemporary mystic, Franklin Merrell-Wolff (1994). An American scientist, mathematician and philosopher of this mid century, and professor at Stanford University, Merrell-Wolff left behind both a diary as a personal record of his own realization of Transcendent Consciousness *(Pathways Through to Space)*, as well as a thorough philosophical and scientific analysis of his realization *("The Philosophy of Consciousness without an Object")*. He used many terms to describe the unfolding of his realization, finding the usual words such as "void", "emptiness", "space", "fullness", "plenum" or "That" as variously unsatisfactory because of their individual potentials for misinterpretation. He used the term "Consciousness-without-an-object" as his main symbol, but eventually he returned to the alternative symbol of "SPACE".

> "... I isolated the subjective moment from the relative manifold of objective consciousness, ... and the result was Emptiness, Darkness, and Silence, i.e., Consciousness with no object."
> (Merrell-Wolff, 1994, p 29).

Of his own Realization, or Recognition, he said:

> "I saw that genuine Recognition is simply a realization of Nothing, but a Nothing that is absolutely substantial and identical with the SELF. ...I found myself at once identical with the Voidness, Darkness, and Silence, but realized them as utter though ineffable, Fullness in the sense of Substantiality, Light, in the sense of Illumination and Sound, in the sense of pure formless Meaning and Value. The deepening of consciousness that followed at once is simply inconceivable and quite beyond the possibility of adequate representation. ...All language as such, is defeated when used as an instrument of portrayal of the transcendent."
> (Merrell-Wolff, 1994, p 263).

Finally the text *Light on the Path* (Collins, 1976) describes the opening of the Centre of Consciousness in metaphorical and poetic terms:

> "Look for the flower to bloom in the silence that follows the storm; not till then. It shall grow, it will shoot up, it will make branches and leaves and form buds, while the storm continues, while the battle lasts. But not till

the whole personality of the man is dissolved and melted – not until it is held by the divine fragment which has created it, as a mere subject for grave experiment and experience – not until the whole nature has yielded and become subject unto its higher self, can the bloom open. Then will come a calm such as comes in a tropical country after the heavy rain, when nature works so swiftly that one may see her action. Such a calm will come to the harassed spirit. And in the deep and silence the mysterious event will occur which will prove that the way has been found. Call it by what name you will, it is a voice that speaks where there is none to speak – it is a messenger that comes, a messenger without form or substance; or it is the flower of the soul that has opened. It cannot be described by any metaphor. But it can be felt after, looked for, and desired, even amid the raging of the storm. The silence may last a moment of time or it may last a thousand years. But it will end. You will carry its strength with you. Again and again the battle must be fought and won. It is only for an interval that Nature can be still. ... seek it by making the profound obeisance of the soul to the dim star that burns within. Steadily, as you watch and worship, its light will grow stronger. Then you may know you have found the beginning of the way. And when you have found the end its light will suddenly become the infinite light."

Collins, 1976, pp 5-7

38. *From the Centre of Consciousness comes the gentle whispering of the Inner Teacher. Love whispers.*

The flow of communication from the Centre of Consciousness is extremely subtle. It is so subtle that doubt is a serious obstacle. A noisy mental field can impair the ability to distinguish the intuitive flow from the normal contents of the mind which obscure that communication. Ultimately the mind must be capable of still, one-pointed concentration. This evolves gradually through the regular and systematic use of the concentration exercises that form the discipline of meditation.

The experience is of a wordless flow of the purest knowing. Initially the phenomenon is intermittent but as the experience of the Centre becomes natural and spontaneous (*sahaja*), then the flow becomes continuous whenever the mind is turned inward and relatively still. The communication flows both ways between the disciple and the Inner Teacher like a quiet, metaphorical whispering. There may be occasional words or sentences, but the communication is usually a wordless flow of pure meaning and understanding.

Sometimes complex concepts are injected into the mind from the Centre as a simultaneous intuitive gestalt. One can sense the presence of this gestalt somewhere deep in the mind in no time and no space. One can access that gestalt at any time and extract from it aspects of its contents for translation into language. A gestalt might encompass a scientific insight, a five-year plan, the deep meanings of a sutra, or a whole musical composition. Science and the arts are full of many such examples. The French mathematician, Henri Poincare, describes how solutions to mathematical problems occurred to him:

> "One evening, contrary to my custom, I drank black coffee and could not sleep. Ideas arose in crowds; I felt them collide until pairs interlocked, so to speak, making a stable combination. By the next morning I had established the existence of a class of Fuchsian functions, those which come from the hypergeometric series; I had only to write out the results, which took but a few hours."
> Ghiselin, 1955, p 36.

There are rich stories about how the glorious music of Handel's Oratorios poured into his mind and through his pen to paper. Here is Mozart's own description of his creative insights:

> "When I am completely myself, entirely alone, and of good cheer ... it is on such occasions that ideas flow best and most abundantly. Whence and how they come, I know not; nor can I force them; nor do I hear in my imagination the parts successively but I hear them all at once. The committing to paper is done quickly enough, for everything is already finished; and it rarely differs on paper from what was in my imagination."
> Mozart

But more than the whisperings of knowledge flow into the mind from the Centre. There are also the whisperings of love - and much more:

Love Whispers

> "It whispers from the heights,
> It whispers from the depths,
> It whispers from the mountains and the streams,
> It whispers from above and from below,
> From the petals of flowers,
>   From my little brooklet's flow.
> It whispers from there and everywhere.
>   Love is a whisper divine.
> But among all the whispers I have ever heard,
> Her whisper is supreme,
>   Fulfilling all my wishes
>   And life's greatest dream."
> Swami Rama, Love Whispers, 1986b, p1

❋

The Warrior Within

39. *In Consciousness the Inner and the Outer Teachers are One and the Same.*

What we have described in the previous section is the Centre of Consciousness, to use Swami Rama's terminology. This is the Inner Teacher or Inner Guru in the yoga tradition.

One of the first things the student learns is that the outer teacher, the physical guru, is but an expression of the Inner Teacher. In consciousness the Inner and the outer teachers are one and the same. Paradoxically the student may learn this through the stimulus of confusion. On the one hand you have the inner experience of the Centre of Consciousness awakening, and on the other you now have the guidance of an outer physical guru. Which do you follow? What is the relationship between the two? When that dilemma becomes focussed, thereby creating the inner thrust of a sincere question, the Centre will answer with an unequivocal inner experience.

One of us had been camping in the mountains and had awakened to a beautiful day. The experience of the spaciousness of the Centre had been very strong. Yet I felt a feeling of frustration and longing for some real answers to the search for inner truth, so much so that I had begun to explore another path and whether I should subscribe to some lessons. Suddenly there was the strong sense of a severe inner scolding. I dropped the book and never looked at it again. The sense of the Presence became very strong, not only within, but also without - impassively watching from everywhere I looked. I drove to a favourite hiking trail and climbed to a mountain lake totally immersed in that Presence. I sat on the rocks by its shore pondering these peculiar events of the day. Again I thought about the puzzle of the two guides, the inner and the outer. Suddenly there was the strong inner sense of Swami Rama as a personality. Then as I watched inside, that "entity" sensed as Swamiji dissolved into the Presence Itself and the two became one. There was a certain intuition and knowing that the two are one and the same.

Communication to the Inner Teacher is communication to the Outer Master and vice versa.
Teaching from the Inner Teacher is teaching from the Outer Master and vice versa.

"You I will teach in Silence!" Swamiji would sometimes say to particular students.

Once during a visit to our Master's ashram one of us wrestled with inner doubt about the veracity of some of these inner experiences because they seemed so subtle. We had not seen Swamiji in person throughout this visit and we were ready to leave early the next morning. As usual we sent our thanks for his hospitality through his secretary. Immediately there was a phone call to our room: "Swamiji will see you both now." As we made our way to his quarters my inner turmoil became acute. Suddenly there was clarity - what was needed was to ask for one's doubts to be removed! He greeted us warmly, and then turned to me and said, "You have a question for me." "Swamiji, please remove my doubts!" I blurted out. He smiled lovingly, asked us about our practices and prescribed some refinements, gave us his blessing and gently sent us on our way. Thereafter neither of us ever had any more doubts about the Centre.

It is this inner link that allows the teaching to flow continuously to the new disciple even though physically the disciple may spend very little direct time in the guru's presence. In deed one soon finds out that those who do the real work and are closest to the master may not be those who physically seem to surround him often.

The space of the Centre is the Now. The Master lives in the Now and what he says must be understood in that way, beyond linear time.

40. *The Voice of the Master is the Voice of the Silence.*

Learning to work with the Centre of Consciousness and through It to the master now becomes the priority for the student. Indeed the master will force the process by deliberately keeping the student at arms length and not responding to questions unless it is clear that the student needs some external input to this learning process. For one day the master will move on and the student must be able to stand alone with certainty in the guidance from the Centre. When pushed into deep water you soon gain the confidence to use what you learned in your swimming lessons in shallow water. The fledgling only learns to fly when the mother robin pushes it out of the nest. But the push only comes when the little bird is ready.

We quote here a powerful excerpt from *Light on the Path* that describes the Centre as the Warrior Within. Read it between the lines with intuition. Although it is metaphorical, it describes exactly how to work with the Centre in real life.

THE WARRIOR WITHIN

"Stand aside in the coming battle, and though thou fightest be not thou the warrior. Look for the warrior and let him fight in thee. Take his orders for battle and obey them. Obey him not as though he were a general, but as though he were thyself, and his spoken words were the utterance of thy secret desires; for he is thyself, yet infinitely wiser and stronger than thyself. Look for him, lest in the fever and hurry of the fight thou mayest pass him; and he will not know thee unless thou knowest him. If thy cry reach his listening ear then will he fight in thee and fill the dull void within. And if this is so, then canst thou go through the fight cool and unwearied, standing aside and letting him battle for thee. Then it will be impossible for thee to strike one blow amiss. But if thou look not for him, if thou pass him by, then there is no safeguard for thee. Thy brain will reel, thy heart grow uncertain, and in the dust of the battle-field thy sight and senses will fail, and thou wilt not know thy friends from thy enemies.

He is thyself, yet thou art but finite and liable to error. He is eternal and is sure. He is eternal truth. When once he has entered thee and become thy warrior, he will never utterly desert thee, and at the day of the great peace he will become one with thee."

Collins, 1976, p9

41. The Inner Ashram has opened.

We hear much about spiritual ashrams and about the challenges of ashram life. But with the opening of the Centre and the realization that It and the master are one in Consciousness, one then learns that there is an Inner Ashram, a kind of inner place in no space and no time where the master and his disciples are one in love, will, wisdom and action. With the opening of the Centre one finds the entry, the portal to that inner space. The qualification for admission is a state of consciousness that the Centre brings and enough mind control not to bring disturbing vibrations - in short, to have found some measure of inner peace, yet another gift from the Centre. Indeed, the Centre makes all things possible in both heaven and earth!

42. Having been tested and found to be qualified, the student is accepted as a disciple. The Inner Teacher has responded with the grace of a Master.

43. The relationship is eternal.

And how the Master will test! - over and over and over, patiently waiting until the student is ready.

We stood with Swamiji one warm evening in the beautiful gardens of his ashram by the Ganges in Rishikesh. There was a full March moon overhead. The fragrance from the flowers was intoxicating. We discussed aspects of the rural health development project we were planning with him for his new hospital. Suddenly he turned to us and holding our eyes forcefully and steadily in his gaze, quietly he said, "Our relationship is eternal!" The master had taken disciples.

> "Ask and it shall be given you;
> Seek, and ye shall find;
> Knock, and it shall be opened unto you."
> Matthew 7:7

> "When the student is ready,
> the Master will appear."

44. The entry to the Path has at last been found.

When experiences of the Centre dawn as described in sutra 36, especially if they are powerful, students may think they are enlightened. They may make the mistake of setting themselves up as "masters", of leaving the Teacher, or of stopping their practices thinking the goal has been reached. Nothing could be further from the truth. Let us illustrate with a metaphor.

Throughout the long night you have stayed awake in preparation for the dawn. Now the time is ripe and you enter the shivery stillness of predawn to wait. As you gaze towards the East you begin to detect the light on the horizon. Faint at first, the glow begins to grow, anticipating the glory to come. There comes a sudden burst of brilliance as the edge of the sun peaks over the horizon. The dawn has come. This is where you are on the Path. The blazing, full brilliance of the sun at noon is yet many hours away. If you felt you were dedicated to the spiritual path before, if you felt you were working hard before, you have merely qualified for the serious work. Now you will feel dedication and effort like never before. Once the light dawns there is no return from the fullness of the day to come.

45. The Centre of Consciousness calls the student to discipleship.

The entry to the Path has at last been found and the student must prepare to tread it with full commitment. For now the Centre of Consciousness calls the student to discipleship. There will come a point when the aspirant will feel the power of that call. Paradoxically the call to discipleship comes from within the student - from the Centre - and not from the outer Master as it may seem. The paradox is resolved when one remembers that the outer Master and the Centre are one and the same in Consciousness, in essential Being. But the student has free will. The student must make the decision to respond, the commitment to answer, to cross over the threshold and to begin to tread the Path.

46. To cross over the threshold the student must die to the world.

47. Total surrender and commitment are required, for the Inner Teacher ultimately is one's own Self.

To answer, to cross over the threshold and to begin to tread the Path, the student must die to the world - be strong enough to leave behind worldly attractions and attachments. Beginning in sutra 79 we will discuss in detail the concept of the identity shift, a shift in self-identity from a small self - an individualized ego - to the large Self, the Spiritual Self. Can you dare to be who you really are? Like oil and water, spirit and the world are qualitatively mutually exclusive. Just as a woman cannot be "a little bit pregnant" one cannot compromise the world and Spirit - have one's cake and eat it too. The commitment is nothing short of total and is irreversible.

That realization will bring the astute student some considerable pause. The world is the centre and spirit is something longed for perhaps, something occasional, something now and then that intrudes in the busy flow of daily life. But one's world will be turned inside out. Spirit will become the Centre and the preoccupation, and all that was so important in daily life will fall away like so much chaff. When the decision is made this process happens automatically under Spirit's direction. It is a death experience, a sequence of repeated deaths, both small and large, as all that the new disciple held dear in the world turns to ashes and falls away before the fire of that Inner Light.

But if the student is not strong enough, not yet ready, the portal will close. For to hesitate is also a decision against. There is no fault. If the aspirant wants to sleep and dream a little longer, all is well. Spirit's patience is infinite. For the portal will close only for awhile to allow the student to strengthen his or her detachment through further worldly experience until he or she tires of the dream. For once the portal has opened the relationship is eternal.

> "Once having passed through the storm and attained the peace, it is then always possible to learn, even though the disciple waver, hesitate and turn aside. The voice of the Silence remains within him, and though he leave the path utterly, yet one day it will resound and rend him asunder and separate his passions from his divine possibilities. Then with pain and desperate cries from the deserted lower self he will return."   Collins, 1976, p23

To answer the call, total surrender, total commitment is required. For the Inner Teacher is ultimately an expression of one's own Self.

III THE CURRICULUM

The First Curriculum

If there is an Inner Teacher, then what is the curriculum? There are some major lessons to be learned by the beginning disciple. Here is a poetic statement of this initial curriculum as found in the text of Light on the Path (Collins, 1976).

"Listen to the song of life.

Store in your memory the melody you hear.

You can stand upright now, firm as a rock amid the turmoil, obeying the warrior who is thyself and thy king. Unconcerned in the battle save to do his bidding, having no longer any care as to result of the battle, for one thing only is important, that the warrior shall win, and you know he is incapable of defeat -- standing thus, cool and awakened, use the hearing you have acquired by pain and by the destruction of pain. Only fragments of the great song, come to your ears while yet you are but man. But if you listen to it, remember it faithfully, so that none which has reached you is lost, and endeavor to learn from it the meaning of mystery which surrounds you. In time you will need no teacher. For as the individual has voice, so has that in which the individual exists. Life itself has speech and is never silent. And its utterance is not, and you that are deaf may suppose, a cry: it is a song. Learn from it that you are a part of the harmony; learn from it to obey the laws of the harmony.

Regard earnestly all the life that surrounds you.

Learn to look intelligently into the hearts of man.

Regard most earnestly your own heart.

For through your own heart comes the one light which can illuminate life and make it clear to your eyes.

Study the hearts of man, that you may know what is that world in which you live and of which you will to be a part. Regard to the constantly changing and moving life which surrounds you, for it is formed by the hearts of man; and as you learn to understand their constitution and meaning, you will by degrees be able to read the larger word of life.

Speech comes only with knowledge. Attain to knowledge and you will attain to speech.

Collins, 1976, pp 11-13

48. *Learn to walk in joy.*

Keys for Contemplation

- **The Ananda aspect of the Centre of Consciousness.**
- **Inexplicable happiness.**
- **Perpetual wonder.**

Walking in joy comes from awareness of the *ananda* (bliss or love) aspect of the Centre of Consciousness. As an initial manifestation of the Self, the Centre shares the essential characteristics of *sat, cit, ananda* - existence, consciousness, and bliss. The disciple experiences an inexplicable joy that bubbles up from within regardless of external circumstances. One is simply and unexplainably happy.

This is indeed the secret of happiness to which all people aspire. It flows from within from the Centre. It is independent of any favourable constellation of external circumstances. Hence the disciple ceases useless efforts to influence or arrange external circumstances to try to make himself or herself happy.

This high vibrational internal state varies from moment to moment in quality. Sometimes it is joy. Sometimes it is a gentle happiness. And other times there is contentment, tranquillity, or peace. All of these are high vibrational states attuned to the Centre of Consciousness. It is the presence of these high internal states that signals one's alignment with the Centre and that one is creating or manifesting appropriately in the external world, as will be discussed in sutras 76 through 87 below. At other times one may experience the influx of powerful inspiration from the energy that creates worlds. Or the Centre may acknowledge an insight with a gentle thrill that passes through the body like a wave of bliss, producing a gentle shivering with goose bumps.

The disciple learns to walk in perpetual wonder, to delight in and marvel at the wonder of creation that surrounds us all. One develops attitudes of praise, gratitude, and reverence. A useful practical exercise is to learn to marvel. Continuously marvel at the wonders of creation and let feelings of praise, appreciation and gratitude flow forth in abundance. This exercise can be particularly effective in the outdoors during a long walk through the beauties of nature. The objective is to invoke a stable, pleasant state of mind, which both facilitates connection to the Centre and also produces coherence in the cardiac and central nervous systems (3).

49. *Learn integrity in all things.*

Keys for Contemplation

- **What you see is what you get.**
  Walk your talk.
- **Align all parts of the personality with the Centre of Consciousness so that there is neither resistance nor inner conflict in thought and action.**
- **Learn to trust the Inner Teacher**
  * How do you know the guidance is correct?
  * Evolving faith.

To think, speak and act with integrity in all things is critical. In the West we have ways of expressing this idea in common speech. "What you see is what you get." "Walk your talk."

Integrity is an aspect of the *yama*, *satya*, or truthfulness. But it goes beyond telling the truth and honesty. The issue here is a clarity of mind in which the grasping of the ego is significantly attenuated. The clarity arises from nonattachment and the mental tranquillity associated with it. The idea of grasping refers to attachment accompanied by the associated positive or negative emotions or feelings characteristic of *raga* or *dvesha*, of attachment or aversion. These constitute two of the *kleshas* or afflictions that cause suffering referred to in the *Yogasutras*, II.3.

Another way of saying the same thing is that because of emotional colouring the awareness as ego has something it wants or desires. It has an agenda. Often that agenda is hidden - sometimes even from the individual. One begins to use manipulation to achieve the agenda; politics and negotiation are born. That is why the ego has been referred to as the "political self". Despite the win-win paradigm for negotiation, this process usually really only results in a win-lose situation. Whatever guidance comes through the Centre now becomes distorted and misdirected by these agendas just as surely as pure white light is coloured by passing through a blue filter to illuminate everything in a distorted wash of blue.

The disciple with integrity is detached and unconcerned with the fruits of his or her action. The concern is only to follow the directive of the spiritual guidance from the Centre as a pure duty to be done for its own sake and in service to that Centre. It is right action; a sense of what is required to be done in any particular situation.

This is selfless service or Karma Yoga. The word "selfless" refers to the egoless or detached nature of the act. It is also service above self. Again the word "self" refers to the ego, and the word "above" implies the Centre of Consciousness. Thus Karma Yoga is action flowing from the Centre of Consciousness. The personality, including the ego, is the instrument of that action. The instrument can only play the role through detachment. The initiation of action actually comes from the Centre. The personality acts as implementor of the guidance given. Yoga is skill in action (Bhagavad Gita II.50). Thus the instrument and the implementation must both be skilled, in addition to there being clarity to the spiritual guidance that flows from the Centre.

Integrity results when all parts of the personality are aligned with the Centre of Consciousness so that there is neither resistance nor inner conflict in thought and action (7).

The disciple must develop a relationship of trust with the Inner Teacher. How does the disciple know that the guidance is correct? The guidance is so subtle, the flow of wisdom such a faint whisper in the beginning, that the disciple will wrestle mightily with doubt. And indeed the master may well address the disciple's doubt specifically. But the ultimate criterion is that the guidance is correct because it works in the world. This is an evidence-based criterion.

Developing a relationship with the Centre of Consciousness is a skill. There are three rules for success. The first is practice. The second is practice. The third is practice! The continuous, unceasing communion and communication with that Presence which is implied in *abhyasa* or *Isvara Pranidhana*, is what is needed to develop this level of skill (see sutras 68 through 75). The relationship evolves gradually over many years, even decades, as the disciple receives the guidance through all of life's exigencies, and learns to trust its correctness.

Faith evolves in the process. Swami Rama used to describe yogic faith as something that evolves from experience, rather than something that is simply believed from authority. One receives some guidance, one follows it, it works in practice, and based on that experience one is willing to follow further guidance. If one can learn to swim in shallow water, then based on that experience one has faith that if one jumps into deep water then one also will be able to swim. Faith in the guidance about small matters leads to faith in the guidance about serious matters of high import and risk. One learns to serve step-by-step: first in little things, and then in big things that have enormous consequence. This is what makes Yoga a spiritual science. By faith we really mean a degree of certainty in a system of belief which would be analogous to hypothesis or theory in science. Such and such is real or so. The degree of our certainty in this belief reflects the degree of our faith that the evidence or experience supporting this belief is so. Yogic faith is evidenced-based faith documented by personal experience of the teachings received from the master or Inner Teacher, rather than blind faith in a belief system or authority.

50. Learn unconditional love.

Keys for Contemplation

- **Love yourself.**
- **Learn generosity.**
- **Use resources to invest in others.**
- **Create evolutionary synergies.**
- **Be a gardener of souls.**
- **Be selfless.**

There is a story told about Rabbi who was a great lover of God (Prakash, 1998). One day a student found him at home in tears. Asked why he was crying the Rabbi said that last night he had had a vision of God. His student was puzzled. How could the Rabbi be so sad if he had been blessed with such a vision? "All my life I have tried to be a good Jew." replied the Rabbi. "I have tried to be like Abraham, like Moses, and like Isaac. All my life I have striven to be like them. But God asked me why I wanted to be like them, like someone else, rather than as he created me. Why had I not striven to be like me? Then I realized I had never really loved myself! I have failed in my spirituality. I have wasted my life. That is why I cry."

When we first met our preceptor, Swami Rama, we asked him what we were to do with all of the people and students that seemed to appear out of nowhere for help and support. His gentle reply was very simple, "Love them all unconditionally." Little did we realize at the time how challenging this would be. For it was only later that we understood the secret of unconditional love. First one must be able to love oneself unconditionally, otherwise we project our self-judgments on to others. Our love for them becomes conditional. But the key to unconditional love is the opening of the Centre of Consciousness from which that love flows combined with the creation of sufficient detachment both from self and from others to be able to release the need to make judgments.

Love is a difficult concept in the West. People mean many different things by it. It can describe desire, or infatuation, or the passion of sexuality, and most commonly it reflects attachment. In all such cases the resulting relationship is conditional, a negotiated contract - whether this is conscious or not. If certain conditions are met in the relationship then one can be loving. But love fundamentally flows from the *ananda* aspect of the *saccidananda* that is the Self and the Centre of Consciousness. It may be experienced as bliss, or as a sense of connection or belonging. There is a feeling of oneness, of unification in the relationship.

Swami Rama was the most loving being we have ever experienced. Our memories of him are many and they are all positive, joyful and loving (for he passed through *mahasamadhi* in 1996). He taught us that love in action means giving, generosity, and he taught this through his own behaviour. He was the epitome of generosity and giving.

With the opening of the Centre the disciple learns how to use resources which come into his or her hands to uplift and to help others. Every opportunity becomes a chance to participate in the unfolding of another. One learns to create evolutionary synergies. Here the function of the whole is greater than the function of its parts, and the people who participate in the synergy grow, expand and are spiritually transformed as a result of their participation. The 10 years that we spent with Swamiji helping to create a rural development program as part of a hospital project that he was constructing near Rishikesh in India was the highlight of our lives. It taught us the value of and how to create evolutionary synergies as a way to do Karma Yoga. One learns to delight in seeing others unfold - a friend, a child, a student. One becomes a gardener of souls.

> "The disciple who has the power of entrance, and is strong enough to pass each barrier, will, when the divine message comes to his spirit, forget himself utterly in the new consciousness which falls on him. If this lofty

contact can really rouse him, he becomes as one of the divine in his desire to give rather than to take, in his wish to help rather than be helped, in his resolution to feed the hungry rather than to take manna from Heaven himself. His nature is transformed, and the selfishness which prompts man's actions in ordinary life suddenly deserts him."

Collins, 1976, pp 71-72

51. *Learn the lesson of surrender.*

Keys for Contemplation

- **Surrender to the Centre is total.**
    * **No secrets.**
    * **No appointments.**
    * **No personal space.**
- **The Presence does not judge.**
    * **Infinite patience.**
- **Commitment gradually becomes total.**
- **There is no loss, but rather, gain of freedom.**
    * **Complete freedom can be terrifying.**

There are no secrets from the Centre of Consciousness. There is a story told about a spiritual master who gave an object to each of three disciples and then asked them to go out and hide the objects where they could never be found. After some hours the first disciple returned flushed with success. He assured his master that he had hidden his object where no one could ever find it. He had gone into the woods where there were many wonderful places to hide things. "You have done what was asked." said the master. After another hour the second disciple returned to boast how he had gone to the desert to find a special place to hide his object. Anyone would think to go to the woods to hide something, but no one would ever think to look in the barrenness of the desert.

A long time passed but the third disciple did not appear. Everyone became concerned. Just as the master was about to send someone to search, the third disciple entered the room, walking slowly and appearing down cast. He approached his master with hesitation, and handed back his object. Sternly the master asked him, "Have you failed to carry out my command?" Sadly the disciple acknowledged his failure. "Sir, I could not find a hiding place. When I looked in a tree I realized I was being watched. When I looked under a stone I was still being watched. No matter where I went or what I did, I could never get away from the feeling that I was being watched. Sir, I have failed." The master smiled lovingly at the disciple and said, "On the contrary, you are the only one who passed the test."

As the Centre opens and as its Presence becomes more and more stable and continuous, however dim, the disciple learns that he or she must surrender all to that constant Witness. One does not work with the Inner Teacher by appointment: during this time I will work with You, but this other time is for me and please go away! The Presence is eventually total. It observes your most intimate and embarrassing moments in every waking second, and eventually even in dreaming and sleep. The surrender of your personal space is total. It takes a strong and balanced personality to withstand this continuous scrutiny as well as some degree of detachment and purification through living out the *yamas* and *niyamas*. One can imagine that if one's physical master were present observing one's practices, for example, one would be giving them extra attention and effort. Imagine then the impact on the one's behaviour that results from the presence of the continuous Witness! One's thought word and deed are inspired to new heights!

Fortunately the Presence does not judge no matter what you may think, say or do. The Centre is infinitely patient, endlessly and unconditionally loving. It is always ready to proceed when you are. Eventually the disciple learns through surrender to do all things enveloped in the secure, ever loving, and infinitely tolerant unconditional love of that Presence. It is this experience that helps the disciple to learn unconditional love of self and others.

And so the disciple's obedience gradually becomes total, as bit by bit over a long time he or she surrenders boundaries, expectations, desires, beliefs, rules, structures, attachments, likes and dislikes - everything. Through surrender there is a complete deconstruction of the disciple's model of the world with release of the attached consciousness bound into the ego so it can shift its identification to the Centre.

For a considerable time the disciple will puzzle over the issue of free will. The ego consciousness will feel that it is losing its freedom by having to surrender to this separate, albeit higher, Centre of Consciousness. It will feel keenly the loss of its separateness and its personal space. For it carries the traditional belief that freedom means doing your own thing, regardless of any impact on others or on the environment. But that separation from the Centre is what causes pain and suffering, ignorance of the consequences of doing your own thing. In actual fact the surrender releases your free will rather than binds it, by dissolving all of the external and psychic structural context and conditioning that forms your model of the world and your ego, your self-identity, and that limits you. Eventually you realize that, in fact, the obedience is not to "another", but to your own true Self. It is the ego that is the "other". If the initial paradox of subject-object consciousness in which the Self seems to know Itself as an object can be accepted, one realizes that the flow of wisdom comes from one's true Self which is freedom. The ego consciousness is the true bondage.

At this point the disciple discovers that complete freedom is terrifying! If you could do anything, have anything, and have any possible resource with no requirements or demands, no shoulds or oughts, then what would you do? What would you want? What would you do with your life? Most of us do not face that challenge because our karma creates ongoing life experiences that carry us along, immersing us in the details of everyday demands and living. But if suddenly all of that stopped, what would you do with your time? You might ask, "What is my mission? What is the purpose of my life?" Then you would receive the surprising answer, "You can do whatever you want to do." That kind of freedom to choose can be terrifying. Mastership carries a heavy responsibility. In this situation, despite our complaining, most of us run back to the crutch of those psychic supports and limitations of one's model of the world rather than try to face the terror of that challenge. It is like the young child who has learned to stand and then to walk hanging on to furniture and walls for support. The terror of letting go of all of these supports must be faced to be able to walk upright alone. If the soul is to spread its wings and fly there comes a time when it must leap out of the nest. Each of us must walk the spiritual path alone. The Inner Teacher is only a guide.

52. Learn that wherever you go, you carry the Light within.

Keys for Contemplation

- **Become a helpless healer and uplifter.**
  * **Accept that responsibility.**
- **Learn respect for that influence.**
- **Being a spiritual guide evolves naturally.**
- **The source of talent and genius.**

By the Light, of course, one means the Centre of Consciousness. That Light is capable of influence wherever you go and in whatever situation you may find yourself. Your very presence in that situation can be healing and uplifting. You need do nothing, you cannot help it. It becomes who and what you are. It now becomes hard to hide your light under a bushel! So become a helpless healer, a helpless uplifter. Accept that responsibility with humility.

As you experience Its effects, you learn profound respect for that influence. On occasion you will meet the rare individual in whom the Centre has opened. There will be an instant mutual recognition with only the passage of a very few words. It is as though one light worker meets another in the daily round of duties with a passing acknowledgement of mutual respect.

In these days of the new millennium with all the long-awaited prophecies imminent, one hears a great deal about being a spiritual counsellor. In the context of the Centre of Consciousness, being a spiritual guide simply evolves naturally. One cannot help but become a spiritual guide of some kind. Others recognize that there is something special about you, that you have some kind of wisdom. They will seek you out informally even though they may not know what it is that they sense about you. You will find yourself supporting and uplifting others. And if you have acquired the skills of counselling and therapy professionally then your impact and power will increase immeasurably.

It is also worth noting that the intuition from the Centre can spark the genius of talent in all fields of human endeavour.

53. *Learn to live with high inner energy flows.*

Keys for Contemplation

- **The awakening by *shaktipat*.**
- **The descending Bliss.**
- **Living with precision.**
- **Divinization of the personality.**
- **Coordinating the *koshas*.**

If the disciple has a relationship with a physical master, then the awakening of the Centre or its intensification may follow on initiation by *shaktipat* from the master. Subsequently one learns gradually to adapt to and to live with increasing, and at times enormous flows of energy through the personality.

The disciple becomes able to appreciate a descending force from that Centre. It may come at times like a bliss that the body can endure only for short periods. As these energies rise and fall one's *sadhana*, one's spiritual practices and lifestyle, become very precise. Great care is needed with diet, exercise and sleep to maintain balance. Diet is particularly stressed in advanced texts on practice (Swami Rama, 1986a). Swami Rama used to speak of the four urges: food, sex, sleep, and self- preservation. The latter refers to what we commonly call stress. Regulation of all of these urges becomes very precise and important. They are to the physical level what the disciplines of moral behaviour are to the psychological realm.

Rather than an intellectual process requiring memorization or the use of contemplation and rationality, the process is more like the training of an Olympic athlete, or a concert pianist or a highly skilled surgeon. These individuals think nothing of practising 8 to 10 hours a day and undertaking a course of training that may last as long as 15 years. Yet surprisingly, we are not prepared to put similar effort into our *sadhana*. The results of this prolonged and gradual process is that the personality is slowly transformed, divinized, casting off impurities at all levels as it goes. The process can be demanding and is not always pleasant.

The Mother, who was Sri Aurobindo's partner, described the need for all layers of the personality to "catch up" as one forges ahead in this process. Each surge of energy, each step on the Path has to be integrated fully into manifestation and expression through the personality. This process of integration is experienced as a plateau in one's progress. As soon as the integration is complete then one moves to the next higher plateau. If the different layers of the personality become too out of phase during this process, then illness can result. The Mother and Aurobindo called this yogic illness (The Mother, 1979).

> "If you're doing meditation correctly, you're in for some very rough and frightening times. Meditation as a 'relaxation response' is a joke. Genuine meditation involves a whole series of deaths and rebirths; extraordinary conflicts and stresses come into play. All of this is just barely balanced by an equal growth in equanimity, compassion, understanding, awareness, and sensitivity, which makes the whole endeavour worthwhile."
> Comments from an interview with Ken Wilber.
> Combs, 1995, p231.

54. Learn the art of intuition. Herein lies the seed of Jnana Yoga.

Keys for Contemplation

- **Intuition is the direct perception of Truth. The mind is used as a "sixth" sense.**
- **Language is unnecessary for thought.**
- **Language is an inadequate representation of intuition.**
- **The mind, indeed all of the universe of energy, is a perfect <u>process</u>, and not a <u>thing</u>. There is no place in a process for NOW.**
- **To live truly in the NOW is to live beyond time, space and causation in the eternal Centre of Consciousness.**

Mastering intuition is key to working with the Centre of Consciousness. The process is both an art and a skill. It comes gradually from long practice and training. The whisperings of intuition are available to us all. But in Western culture we confuse intuition often with instinct. Moreover, the tyranny of reason persuades us to dismiss intuition as unreliable. Although scientists would never admit, in fact the march of real discovery in science is led by intuition with the rational faculty working out the practical implications of the insights given.

With true intuition one gains a direct perception of Truth. The mind is used as though it were a sixth sense. The Truth is perceived directly without any intervention of language, reasoning or calculating in the same way that physical reality is perceived directly by the five physical senses. In a particular context one simply knows instantly and directly what needs to be known.

One is surprised to learn that language is not necessary for knowing or thinking. This is contrary to current scientific thought and popular belief, which hold that one needs language to think. Intuitive knowing is holistic and instantaneous. It may come as a continuous gentle flow of knowing or as an injection of knowledge into the mind as an instantaneous gestalt which can be accessed over and over for its rich content. One soon learns that language is a clumsy and inadequate representation of such a gestalt and much too slow. It cannot capture all of the knowledge nor can it capture its richness.

One learns to realize that the mind is a subtle energy field, and indeed all the universe of energy, is not a thing. Rather, it is a perfect process. Through ignorance one may use the process to create for good or ill. But whatever the result, the process for manifesting it always works perfectly.

There is no place in a process for Now. The ego lives as a structure in time, space and causation. The desires and agendas of the "political self" which is the ego, can exist in time since they live in the future based on the past.

Technically, where is "now" in time? One can delineate a narrow segment on the time line and call it now. Yet that segment has a beginning and an end, however small its length. Indeed, one can cut finer and finer segments on that line of time to try to collapse the future and the past into a limit of "now." At the limit this process results in an infinitesimal point designating "now" that is but an imaginary concept.

The position of Now in a process, rather, lies outside the flow of the process as a point of observation. The observer is the Centre of Consciousness which exists beyond time in the transcendent, eternal Now. It introjects its revelations into the process and flow that is mind in the realm of time, space and causation.

It is very popular to talk about living in the present and in the now. People misunderstand and struggle to keep their awareness focussed in the present time. The true meaning of this concept comes only with the opening of the Centre of Consciousness. The Centre of Consciousness is the eternal Now. For one's primary self-identity to lie in that Centre means to experience an eternal Now outside the flow of time, space and causation. This is to live in the eternal Now or Presence and to have its infinite power available in the moment. To live truly in the Now is to live beyond time, space and causation in the eternal Centre of Consciousness.

55. *Intuition is the Voice of the Silence.*

Keys for Contemplation

- **Distinguish intuition from all other mental content.**
  - **Learn how the mind constructs your experience.**
- **Avoid the traps of specialness and the psychic.**
- **Intuition is the whispering of a flow of pure knowing into a detached, still mind field.**
  - **The Voice of the Silence.**
  - **"Love Whispers."**
- **Spirit communicates through subtle "feelings".**
  - **Learn to read subtle energy fields.**

One must learn to distinguish the flow of intuition from "everything else", the contents within the mind. That "everything else" lies in time, space and causation. Intuition, however, comes from the Centre of Consciousness beyond, but it is introduced as content into the spatiotemporal energy field of mind.

What are these contents? They are rich and complex. They include an almost infinite range of feelings, which must be distinguished from emotions arising from the subtle body. They include the kinesthetics produced by the neuromuscular structures of the physical body. They include all of the imagery that comes from the five physical senses. In this regard, it is helpful for the student to learn about the modalities, and submodalities that characterize sensual imagery as well as concepts such as sensory dominance, the sequencing of internal imagery in strategies, eye and body accessing cues, etc., as described in a discipline such as Neuro-Linguistic Programming (Cameron-Bandler, 1985; O'Conner and Seymour, 1990).

Other content would include thoughts which often occur as internal dialogue. The products of reason must also be distinguished. One must particularly avoid the common process of post hoc rationalization. So much of human action flows from instinct, habit and conditioning as a reaction to stimuli arising from a certain context. In other words action is so often simply reaction. These conditioned responses act so quickly and below the conscious awareness that they are barely noticed. Then the rational faculty rapidly comes into play to provide a reason for the behaviour. The latter occupies awareness to the exclusion of the former and the individual genuinely feels that he or she has acted rationally when in fact the action has come from conditioning or instinct.

There are other mental contents which must be distinguished that play out their action in time. They include memory and particularly material coming up from the unconscious and subconscious minds, as well as imagination and related states such as reverie or conscious dreaming. One must also become familiar with altered states such as trance, dream, sleep, etc.. None of these constitute the whisperings of intuition and one must learn to distinguish.

It is useful for the student to have good maps of the mind as well as its content and structures which here we call models of the world. It helps to know how the mind constructs experience. Again Neuro-Linguistic Programming and related disciplines can provide useful material such as the meta- and Milton models, models for rapport, or metaprograms (the Meyers-Briggs and Jungian typologies are examples). The Sufi Enneagram system can also be very useful.

But do not go astray. Do not accept visions of guru, gods and goddesses telling you that you are the chosen one with the mission to save the world. If you hear voices in your head then you need to see a psychiatrist. Rather the communications are so subtle that your major battle will be with doubt.

The process involves moving from the subtle, to the subtler, and then to the subtlest. A story is often told of how a bride groom tries to show his bride the star arundhati. It lies in near the pole star. When the pole star is identified the groom then uses it to help his bride find a subtler star next to it. That in turn is used to allow the bride to identify the star arundhati, which by itself is so faint that it would be difficult to identify directly. To hear the whisperings of the Centre of Consciousness one needs a detached and still mind. This is hardest to obtain in the middle of the battle of life when those whisperings are most needed.

What are these whisperings like? They are not like any of the contents of the normal mind noted above. There is no reason, no imagery, nothing to infer, and nothing to figure out. The experience is closest to a flow of pure knowing into the mind. There is no language, although at times a few words may appear.

108 Sutras of the Inner Teacher

The source is the Presence, the Centre of Consciousness. Sometimes there is an instantaneous, total gestalt that seems to sit high in the mind field like a wispy cloud of energy existing in no space and no time. It would take books of language to portray the content of this intuition, and yet its full meaning would still be inadequately expressed. You simply know, and you know that you know, and you know with absolute certainty that what you know is true.

Swami Rama often emphasized the self-evident knowing and certainty of such intuitions. There may be glimpses of direct perceptions such as clairvoyance. The psychologist may have instant and direct perception of an individual's life history and problems without asking. The physician may know intuitively a patient's diagnosis. The writings of Barbara Brennan describe the remarkable insights that can be received from intuitive diagnosis (Brennan, 1987). Swami Rama was a master of intuitive diagnosis. Indeed, one can know anything that one needs to know. One simply needs to ask and to be able to "hear" the response. But "need to know" is the operative phrase here; idle curiosity draws a blank.

One learns that spirit communicates through subtle feelings, and sometimes emotions if strong guidance is needed. Energy fields carry information in their vibrations. Communications from spirit are sensed as subtle feelings, "vibes" in popular language. We normally have many internal states that are sensed the same way. We know we are secure because of how we feel. We know we are free because of a feeling. So one learns to read the meaning of subtle transmissions of feeling, of subtle vibratory energy fields.

"What is Truth? A difficult question; but I have solved it for myself by saying that it is what the 'voice within' tells you."
Mahatma Gandhi

56. One becomes a spiritual guide spontaneously.

Keys for Contemplation

• **How to be a spiritual guide:**
   Channel the Centre of
   Consciousness in all things.
   Follow Spirit without hesitation.
      BUT
   Be a skilled instrument.
   Stay grounded.

❂

In this day of new age writing the student will have heard of channelling. Individuals who have this ability to channel consciously learn to translate into language the ongoing subtle energy transmissions that come to them from the channelled source in the form of whole blocks of meaning and knowing. Effectively what we are talking about here is channelling the Centre of Consciousness in all things: in teaching, studying and reading; in action, writing and speech. This is truly what makes one a spiritual guide. But the instrument, the personality, must be skilled and well-grounded.

> "Until the first step has been taken in this development, this knowledge, which is called intuition with certainty, is impossible to man. And this positive and certain intuition is the only form of knowledge which enables a man to work rapidly or reach his true and high estate, within the limit of his conscious effort. To obtain knowledge by experiment is too tedious a method for those who aspire to accomplish real work; he who gets it by certain intuition, lays hands on its various forms with supreme rapidity, by fierce effort of will; as a determined workmen grasps his tools, indifferent to their weight or any other difficulty which may stand in his way. He does not stay for each to be tested -- he uses such as he sees are fittest."
> Collins, 1976, p34

This little manual, *Light on the Path* (Collins, 1976), has much more to say about the importance of the development of intuition. It emphasizes that the development of intuition in no way disparages the scientific method. The latter is applicable only to matter and to the physical universe. The advance of scientific understanding and technology is a major accomplishment of this century and before. But intuitive knowledge is an entirely different thing. It is not acquired, but rather is more like a faculty of the divine soul, a manifestation of the Centre of Consciousness. It is up to the student to gain awareness of this intuitive faculty by a resolute effort of indomitable will. In this regard faith plays a key role. The engine of faith can accomplish all things. It is like a covenant between the Centre of Consciousness and the ego in the personality. Faith is necessary to obtain intuitive knowledge, for a student must believe that such knowledge exists before he or she can claim and use it.

Simply put: without intuition the student is lost! In the West we worship rationality and the intellect. There is no doubt that these are powerful tools - witness our science and technology. Unfortunately, however, any position can be rationalized or argued. It takes intuition to show what needs to be given to the tools of rationality to bring it into manifestation. Even though it is ridiculed and confused with instinct, good science uses intuition first.

One of us had the good fortune to do a PhD at a prominent North American scientific institute in the early 1970s. At that time there were more Nobelists on faculty than in any other comparable institute worldwide. But despite their scientific brilliance we could not help but be impressed how often some of these highly intelligent people made a mess of their lives and made the lives of their students and colleagues miserable. As a human endeavour, science is as political as any.

57. Learn to be selfish! Share what you have been given that you may receive more.

Keys to Contemplation

- **There is a duty to share knowledge.**
- **Specialness is the teacher's trap.**

The power of intuition grants the gift of speech. By speech we mean the ability to share knowledge, to teach, and the imperative to do so. The gift of speech means the ability to share real knowledge, not just what has been gleaned from books and from others, however well assimilated. The student learns the test for real knowledge. Does the person who is speaking or writing "Know"? If not, then do not waste your time over them. Needless to say, this can substantially reduce one's reading load!

One examines two books. One book is a work of art in design, while the other is rather plain. One is richly written displaying great philosophical skill, while the other is laid out in faltering English. Just holding each of the books and browsing quickly through each in turn is enough to know that despite its unappealing exterior only the author of the plain book "Knows". Not all books can be judged by their cover; nevertheless, some good books have excellent bindings.

Spend your time with the author who Knows and read that book with the intuitive sense from the Centre of Consciousness, enjoying it with deep contemplation. The power of intuition grants this knowledge. And so it will be also with teaching communicated by lecture or by any other medium. But to receive this intuition one must be able to "listen" internally with a still mind coupled with the intent to receive.

With discipleship comes the duty to share knowledge. Truly we teach what we most need to learn ourselves. With intuitive knowledge comes the power of speech. And with this the new disciple finds himself or herself in state of unfolding, of blossoming. There is now the power and the right to demand contact with the divinest element of that state of consciousness into which the disciple has entered - the Centre of Consciousness:

> "But he finds himself compelled, by the nature of his position, to act in two ways at the same time. He cannot send his voice up to the heights where sit the gods till he has penetrated to the deep places where their light shines not all. He has come within the grip of an iron law. If he demands to become a neophyte, he at once becomes a servant. Yet his service is sublime, if only from the character of those who share it. For the masters are also servants; they serve and claim their reward afterwards. Part of their service is to let their knowledge touch him; his first act of service is to give some of that knowledge to those who are not yet fit to stand where he stands. This is no arbitrary decision, made by any master or teacher or any such person, however divine. It is a law of that life which the disciple has entered upon. ... In some confused and blurred manner the news that there is knowledge and a beneficent power which teaches is carried to as many men as will listen to it. No disciple can across the threshold without communicating this news, and placing it on record in some fashion or other."
> Collins, 1976, p 69 - 70.

But in taking up this important task of teaching the new disciple must avoid specialness - the teacher's trap. The spiritual teacher becomes rapidly isolated from meaningful feedback that would allow him or her to grow and to remain balanced. Students adore their teachers, and teachers in their turn can succumb to the glamour and become puffed up with the self-importance of their supposed station and mission. They may be tempted by power and sex. In the Himalayan Tradition this phenomenon has been humorously called "swami worship". People are hesitant to criticize a spiritual teacher's actions. Although those actions may engender much private gossip, the teacher will be the last to hear, if at all. Thus corrective feedback to the teacher is lost, and soon even the teacher can become lost. An egotistical teacher with unquestioning and adoring students, both of whom have lost discrimination, together can create a cult. Swami Rama insisted that students ask hard questions and challenge all teachings with respect. Only knowledge from experience is ultimately reliable. Again *Light on the Path* addresses the problem beautifully:

> "He stands horror-struck at the imperfect and unprepared manner in which he has done this [teach]; and then comes the desire to do it well, and with the desire to help others comes the power. For it is a pure desire, this which comes upon him; he can gain no credit, no glory, no personal reward by fulfilling it. And therefore he obtains the power to fulfill it. ... History ... shows very plainly that there is neither credit, glory, or reward to be gained by this first task which is given to the neophyte. Mystics have always been

sneered at, and seers disbelieved; those who have had the added the power of intellect have left for posterity their written record, which to most men appears unmeaning and visionary. ... The disciple who undertakes the task, secretly hoping for fame or success, to appear as a teacher and apostle before the world, fails even before his task is attempted, and his hidden hypocrisy poisons his own soul, and the souls of those he touches. He is secretly worshipping himself, and this idolatrous practice must bring its own reward."

Collins, 1976, p 71.

One should remind the reader that a consequence of the opening of the Centre of Consciousness is to always carry that Light within. In that state one cannot but influence others in some positive way. Thus one becomes a teacher by default, a spiritual guide spontaneously. In this setting the major teaching comes through role modelling and occurs quite naturally. Information may be passed to the student by oral discourse or on the written page, but the teacher himself or herself is the major teaching. This selfless process stands in contradistinction to the ego and ambition of the above scenario.

"He who thinks himself holier than another, he who has any pride in his own exemption from vice or folly, he who believes himself wise, or in any way superior to his fellow man, is incapable of discipleship. A man must become as a little child before he can entered into the kingdom of heaven."

Collins, 1976, p82

The mystic Persian poet Jelaluddin Rumi told about a young man who had a problem and wanted to find a wise person. A bystander informed him that no one with intelligence lived in the town except for the man over there playing with the children. With some difficulty the seeker got the Sheikh to stop playing long enough to carry on a short conversation. The Sheikh's wisdom was obvious and the seeker eventually asked him why he hid his intelligence. The Sheikh replied that the people wanted to put him in charge, to interpret all the texts and to act as judge and magistrate. But his Inner Knowing only wanted to enjoy Itself. He told the seeker that he was at the same time both a plantation of sugar cane and enjoying the sweetness. He said that acquired knowledge was not like this. It acted instead as bait for popularity, for those who had it worried incessantly whether others liked it or not.

58. Learn the art of conscious death.

Keys for Contemplation

- Part of the curriculum for *vanaprastha*.
- The signs of immanent death.
- Learn to live life as a preparation for death.

One day our teacher was asked about the yogic concept of death. His reply was startling: "Death? I don't recognize the existence of such a thing as death! Change the garments - that's death! We're all just waiting to be reborn. No such thing as ceasing to be. Death is just new birth, rebirth, freedom, liberty, a gateway to eternity!" Needless to say, he now had a rapt and attentive audience!

He then asked to see as many Western books on death as could be found. After reviewing them he said, "Take them all back. There's not a word on death here! Not one single book on death! Oh, there are very good books on grief, on handling the emotional problems attendant on death, on training nurses and doctors to relieve the pain and distress of illness. All of these are good. But there's nothing here on death!"

He then introduced the Tibetan Book of the Dead (The Bardo Thödel), the Kathopanishad from the Vedantic tradition and the Egyptian Book of the Dead, all as examples of books that deal with death itself. He then allowed that perhaps books on near death experiences might be relevant. A near death experience is not true initiatory death in yoga, but is strikingly similar. One finds oneself floating above the physical body in an operating room or after a serious accident or cardiac arrest, and hears the doctors saying you have just died. You watch as they resuscitate you. Then you come back and astonish them by telling them what you heard and saw. A near death experience is similar to some of what is described in the Tibetan Book of the Dead, which, however, goes much further. In a near death experience one goes only a little way into the first Bardo and then comes back.

There ensued some remarkable teachings on death as known in the meditative tradition of yoga (Arya, 1979b; Easwaran, 1992; 1996; Evans-Wentz, 1960; Freemantle and Trungpa, 1975; Swami Rama, 1976; 1996). The topic is an alternative way to express the spiritual dimension in health and healing, and is an essential component of the pursuit of inner health. Here we will touch briefly on a few of those teachings for they are part of the curriculum of *vanaprastha*, the forest dweller (8).

Their essence is twofold. One is the immortality of the Self, the infinite existence of the Spiritual Being which we all are, that Centre of Consciousness.

> "What is not, shall never be
> What is, shall never cease to be ..."
> Bhagavad Gita II.16

The other is that the body is considered to be a garment to be cast off when it wears out.

> "As one removes old garments
>   and puts on new ones,
> So does the master of the body
>   take off the worn flesh
> To wear the new one."
> Bhagavad Gita II.22

Life is a preparation for death. The Greek lawgiver, Solon the Great, stated that only by the way a man ends his life would we know if he has had a successful life. The success of life cannot be measured while someone is still in the process of living. Death becomes the measure of life. By how we die will we know if we have had a fulfilling and happy life. Death is the culmination of life; all the rest is just means. So make life a preparation for death.

> "While this body is yet free of disease,
>   And the old age is yet far away,
> While the strength in the senses yet waxes,
>   And the lifespan is not in ebb,
> The wise man must right now undertake
>   Endeavours for spiritual uplifting,
> For, what effort to dig a well
>   When the house is already on fire?"
> The Puranas

Death becomes an incentive. Accomplish with this body as much as you can of virtue, of something meritorious, of something unselfish. Give as much as you can of yourself and continue to give to God and to your fellow beings. You make a living by what you get, but you make a life by what you give.

> "Earn merit daily as though
> Death holds one by the hair."
> The Laws of Manu

Live a life of basic discipline, a life of unselfishness, a life in which one has fulfilled one's karma, a life in which one has received and given of unselfish love, a life which has not been built around contracts that are entered into and broken at convenience, a life in which there have been permanent relationships where one has dared to commit oneself to persons, to ideals, to a central mission over long periods of time. Thereby you gather the power of thought and learn something of the conscious control of the body, its fields of energy, and its states of awareness. Even though because of the force of karma you cannot avert the hour of death, you can take a certain control over the process. You can sit up, give direction to your thoughts, and die with the name of God on your lips. This is within everyone's reach.

At one time one of the tests of Christian theology was whether a doctrine could lead one to apotheosis (deification, becoming one with God) - to be born a human being, one with this body, but to die a Being of Light, one with God. There could be no more blessed human life than that. But you have to work for that!

> "When you were born you cried
> and the whole world rejoiced.
> Live such a life that when you die
> the whole world cries and you rejoice!"

59. *Learn the importance of positive thoughts and emotions.*

Keys for Contemplation

- **Negativity must be dispelled through constant mindfulness.**
- **The butterfly effect through the law of attraction.**
- **Emotional tone (vibrational signal) determines what manifests and signals alignment with the Centre.**
- **The mind is a creation machine with no off switch!**
- **Never allow yourself the indulgence of entertaining negative thoughts.**

Learn the importance of maintaining positive thoughts and emotions in the mind always. The mind must be constantly watched and no negative thinking allowed. Negativity drops the personality's vibration rate until it is too low to access the Centre of Consciousness, which then disappears from awareness. There are several sutras in the *Yogasutras* that address this issue directly:

> "The mind becomes purified by the cultivation of feelings of amity, compassion, goodwill and indifference respectively towards happy, miserable, virtuous and sinful creatures."
> Yogasutras I.33

These are the four *parikarmas* or purifications in yoga. In Buddhism they are called the *brahma-viharas* or frolicking in God. Their purpose is to purify the mind to make it pleasant and permanently stable so that one-pointedness becomes its natural state.

> "When these restraints (yamas) and observances (niyamas) are inhibited by perverse thoughts, the opposites should be thought of."
> Yogasutras II.33

Again this sutra points to the importance of holding positive thoughts in the mind. The nature of the positive thoughts is described by the traditional restraints and observances of Raja Yoga. It is important to hold in the mind what is desired, rather than what is not desired. When you are asked not to think of a pink elephant, a pink elephant promptly appears in the mind! The unconscious mind does not understand the word "not". It only understands what is pointed to.

The Bhakti Sutras (Prakash, 1998) also deal with the same issue:

43. "Negative companionship should be fully relinquished."

44. "Negative companionship is the cause of selfish desire, anger, delusion, forgetting one's spiritual goal, loss of discrimination, and the loss of everything worthwhile."

In other words one loses direct awareness of the Centre of Consciousness and is left on one's own floundering in the flood. These sutras refer to more than keeping companionship with the wrong people. At a subtle level they refer to companionship of one's thoughts and feelings, not just the companions one keeps in the external world which are a reflection of those thoughts and feelings.

45. "A swelling ocean is raised from the small waves of companionship."

This refers to what might be called the law of attraction. A few negative thoughts in the mind tend to attract more like negative thoughts due to the ways in which the mind links thoughts through association. These negative thoughts, in turn, attract more negative thoughts, which attract more negative thoughts, and so on. The resulting chain reaction soon becomes a flood of negativity that overwhelms the mind and mood. This is analogous in chaos theory to the butterfly effect. The fluttering of the wings of a butterfly over Hong Kong can affect the patterns of storm fronts over New York the next day. This metaphor refers to the sensitivity to initial conditions that is seen in the equations describing chaos.

This is about more than just feeling bad. It has practical implications for karma. The tone of your emotional state and desires determines what manifests, what will be your experience of the world. By emotional tone we refer to the vibrational signal emitted by the personality. Recall that the personality is an energy configuration of many layers suffused with consciousness. All energies carry information and vibrate at some frequency. The energy configuration which is the personality is no exception. We continuously broadcast a vibrational signal to the universe. In metaphorical terms the universe responds to that vibrational signal from moment to moment, to the information it contains related to desire and intent, and then responds by rearranging itself to match the pictures of reality or models of a world which determined the desire. These pictures of reality describe the system of beliefs, values, etc. that has been constructed by the intellect in an ongoing way to allow us to make meaning of our experience and the world (sutra 22). This acts like a kind of blueprint or filter that determines the quality of the vibrational signal representing emotional tone that we emit as we go about the business of desiring and acting.

Thus the presence of positive emotions means that one is aligned with the Centre of Consciousness and will be attracting what is wanted. The presence of negative emotions in the mind means a loss of that alignment, and that we will be experiencing what we do not want. In this regard, one must also remember that health is a creation. Never forget that the mind acts like a creation machine with no off switch.

The bottom line is never allow yourself the indulgence of entertaining negative thoughts.

118 Sutras of the Inner Teacher

60. Learn the art of creativity and effective action.

Keys to Contemplation

"**Yoga is skillfulness in action.**"
Bhagavad Gita II.50
• **Do your duty with right action and right timing.**
• **Karma Yoga is right action flowing consciously from the Centre of Consciousness.**
Follow your Centre without wavering.
• **Live your life and "keep it together".**
• **Learn the art of conscious manifesting.**
The laws of karma are the laws of manifesting.

"*Yogah karmasu kaushalam*" is the motto of the Himalayan Institute founded in the United States by Swami Rama, who was a great Karma Yogi. It means, "Yoga is skillfulness in action" (Bhagavad Gita II.50). This is a very important concept in practice. Part of it is to learn what is the right thing to be done in any given situation, regardless of what you are others may want. One simply does the right thing. This is known as doing your duty. When we would express our gratitude to Swamiji his simple reply was, "I'm just doing my duty." We came to realize that this was an impersonal act of service to the Centre of Consciousness and had nothing to do with personalities or implied favouritism. His love was unconditional.

Skilful action refers to the art of being in the right place, with the right people, doing the right thing, at the right time, in the right way. The student will recall chapter 14 of the Bhagavad Gita referring to *tamasic, rajasic* and *sattvic* behaviours (Swami Rama, 1985). Right action is *sattvic* action. Its essence comes from absorption in the Centre of Consciousness. True Karma Yoga is experienced as action flowing with awareness from the Centre of Consciousness. In other words, the will or intent that drives the action has its source in that Centre rather than in the ego. Using a memorable metaphor, this has been called, "following spirit without hesitation" (Alarius, 1989).

In the usual situation action arises from desire from the ego, and the Centre of Consciousness is veiled from awareness. In right action the Centre of Consciousness is the architect while the ego and personality act in service as the project manager and implementor. When this awareness arises then selfless service with renunciation of the fruits of action becomes natural without having to consciously follow these guidelines that describe Karma Yoga. Until then, follow the guidelines. Because conscious Karma Yoga flows from the Centre of Consciousness it does not create karma in the same way that ego-based action does.

Swami Rama was a stunning example of impactful and effective action. He was a planetary figure. Few realize the extent of his influence in so many fields of endeavour in many countries. The student may be absorbed in the Centre of Consciousness, but he or she must still be able to remember his or her telephone number and zip code! In the West we have the saying, "He's so heavenly-minded that he's no earthly good!"

There is another aspect to skilful action. In the West we would use the phrase, "keeping it together." To be able to serve a master and the Tradition with any effectiveness, it is a minimum requirement for the student to be able to conduct his or her own life sufficiently well that the master does not have to spend time bailing the student out of trouble and cleaning up the mess made of things that the student has been given to do. You must be able to stand on your own in everyday life, and be able to make sensible decisions for at least the major issues of life. This is like a young child being able to walk on its own without being dependent on external support. If the student has to plague the master with dependencies ranging from whom I should marry, or what work should I do all the way down to what colour of socks should I buy, then the student is not ready for real work. One can hardly send a child on an errand if it needs support to walk.

We watched so many people waste Swami Rama's time in this way. He was always gracious and helpful. But eventually we realized that the real work was not always being done by those who seemed physically closest to him. We all would like to have an all-powerful divine parent to magically solve all of our problems without our having to do the challenging work of growth ourselves. This belief in a magic bullet for all our problems is endemic in human society. A good example is the often unrealistic expectations that people have of the health care system to magically, quickly and painlessly fix the consequences of an unhealthy lifestyle for which they should be taking personal responsibility. A master will not allow this kind of dependent relationship in any form.

Swamiji was very firm in breaking any tendency to dependency on him by any of his disciples. To do real work one has to learn to function effectively in the world on one's own and to receive the constant guidance from the master through the Inner Teacher. Indeed, this is how Swamiji trained his disciples. He gave them a project of selfless service as a context for them to establish contact with and learn to express and work with the Inner Teacher. Barring a specific need, the disciple was strongly kept at physical arm's length and rarely saw the master in person, and if he or she did, discussion of needs around the project of service was rarely allowed.

Finally, in learning skilful action the student must learn the art of creating or manifesting with the mind, and to do it consciously. Most of our manifesting is unconscious and the result of conditioning and habit. Indeed, most of us are quite unaware of the key role of the mind in creating our experiences. In other words, the student must learn that the laws of karma are in fact the cause and effect laws of manifestation.

61. Accept that the disciple is protected by the Tradition. All is well; it really is!

62. Learn discrimination in all things. Common sense is rather uncommon!

63. Learn to accept responsibility for Who you really are. Claim your power.

Keys for Contemplation

- **A vision of the Centre of Consciousness is the Self seeing Itself through Itself.**
- **Can you truly accept the potential of who you really are?**

A major challenge on this stage of the path is for the disciple to begin to learn to accept responsibility for who she really is. The disciple must claim his power. Awareness of the Centre of Consciousness, even of its earliest manifestation, raises the question of how this process occurs. If that Centre represents who I really am, then why do I see It as an object? Why do I appear to see my Real Self as an object? The phenomenon is really the Self seeing Itself through or by Itself in consciousness. The focus of consciousness is still at the level of the personality, the ego. The ego and personality exist in subject-object consciousness in the realm of space, time and causation. As the ego, consciousness experiences in subject-object consciousness and thus has its initial awareness of the Self as though It were in object. Later, when the ego is transcended, the infinite and transcendental unity of that Centre will become manifest. One might imagine as a model that the Self sees Itself mirrored in the inner face of *buddhi*. Metaphorically it is as though one is looking at Oneself in a mirror.

To use another metaphor it is easy for you to focus your awareness in a body part like your right big toe. You can become so focussed that you are aware of only your toe. If you could imagine an identity shift so that you became that toe (limited your conscious awareness only to the experience of being a toe) and lost awareness of your real and larger you, then you would have a metaphor for separated ego consciousness. If that toe awareness were to then experience the faintest return of awareness of the larger self, it would experience that as an object, as other than "toeness", because the identity shift back to the larger self has not yet occurred. It all has to do with the locus of your identity - where you place the centre of your awareness, your reference point - in the limited ego or back in the true Self.

If this be the case, then can you really accept Who and What you really are? Can you release, surrender or detach your consciousness from its identification with the boundary beliefs in your mental model of the world that define your sense of self, your identity? The *Yoga Vasishtha* points out a peculiar property of Consciousness. Any notion (i.e. belief) held for a time in consciousness manifests (is experienced as real). You are (experience) who you believe you are (what you believe is real about yourself). In other words Consciousness becomes conditioned or "stained" by the notion, much like a pure crystal placed beside a blue object seems to be blue. It only reflects the object; the crystal itself is unaffected.

The metaphors of Consciousness as mirror discussed in sutra 32 are useful here. Unless the Centre has opened enough to provide a reference point for awareness, then letting go of identity boundaries could be very dangerous and result in fear if not insanity, for the awareness is still anchored in the ego. To let go of the experience of the ego would then be tantamount to death. There is in fact no death of true Consciousness, but it still holds the notion of being the limited self and so would experience a death as thought it were real. Fortunately this will not occur until the Centre as Inner Guide becomes available as the permanent and unchanging point of self-identity.

To use another metaphor, the movie is experienced as real as long as one is associated into and identified with the plot. It is only with detachment that one realizes it is only a movie and becomes aware of the projector, light and screen that conjure up the experience.

An exercise can be done to point to the ephemeral nature of self definitions. Choose a partner. Each of you, in turn, walk slowly towards the other who stands still, and try to sense your boundary of personal space. At what distance from the other person do you feel your personal space start to become crowded or violated? You will know that this distance varies with culture. Let your partner do the same with you. Then each of you stand apart and imagine that boundary you have each defined to be a balloon with you standing in the middle. Now each of you imagine blowing up your boundary balloon until it bursts. Let it grow as big as it has to burst, even if it has to be larger than the room or as big as the universe itself. Keep blowing in your imagination until you experience it bursting. The moment it bursts for each of you, then walk slowly towards each other. Now you will both notice that your personal boundaries have disappeared. You each will walk into each other's embrace.

This whole process with the Centre requires a key identity shift which we will discuss in sutras 81 through 84. To make this identity shift one has to be able to accept the possibility of one's own divinity - that one's essential nature is spirit. This realization may conflict strongly with the student's value systems, especially values that have been instilled in the context of conventional religion. In the West, for example, such a thing would be described as blasphemy in some formulations of Christian theology. This can be a very great obstacle to progress. The inability to transcend these beliefs mean that one retains a limited identity in a state of "toeness" - to reuse our metaphor above - and one is not liberated into the larger, unconditioned consciousness.

64. In learning to act from the Centre, use the power of "as if".

Keys to Contemplation

- **When in doubt, act "as if" you were sure and learn from the feedback.**
    * Blame exists only in your own mind.
- **Learning to act from the Centre is like learning to walk.**
    * You fall a lot until you get the hang of it.
- **Refusing to act when unsure is still a decision.**
    * You cannot but act!
- **Distinguish nonaction from watchful waiting.**
    * Timing is everything.

What do you do if you feel unsure about your inner guidance? Make an experiment. Act "as if" you were sure and learn from the feedback. Most of us have a peculiar idea of learning. We have been too influenced by our educational system. We are presented with finished material and expected to memorize it. Taking in information is not the process of learning required here. Working with the Centre of Consciousness is more like learning a skill such as learning to walk or learning to play a musical instrument, or learning a sport. Have you watched a young child try to learn how to walk? In learning to walk, you fall a lot until you get to hang of it. Moreover, the child displays a single-mindedness in attempting to walk until it finally succeeds. So, persistence, concentration, and learning from feedback are important ingredients.

For this process to succeed you must surrender blame. Again we are educated to believe that when we do not reach a goal we are wrong, we have made a mistake, we are to blame. Nothing interferes with effective learning more than this kind of blame frame or belief system. Our spiritual teacher asked us whether when we are driving our car and suddenly we find our brakes are not working, what do we do? Do we let the car coast to the side of the road and then sit and berate ourselves with great guilt, blaming our situation on not providing proper maintenance for the car?

Our teacher noted that coming from the yoga tradition he was unacquainted with the concept of guilt until he came to the West. In western culture we find it inconceivable that someone could not know what guilt is. But the point he made is that blame and guilt are as useless as they are painful. Simply accept the feedback from the incident about the importance of properly caring for your vehicle, have the car towed and the brakes fixed, and get on with your journey. The key is to learn from the experience and not be immobilized by feeling bad or guilty about it.

Thus learning to work with the Centre of Consciousness means making lots of mistakes, or more correctly, receiving much feedback as you refine the process.

It is more like how a missile locks onto its target. The focus is fuzzy to start with, wavering back and forth. But as the feedback starts to come in, the missile's guidance system corrects for the overshoot, refining its focus, until it is locked precisely onto the target.

This kind of learning by feedback characterizes a complex physical skill. But it can also apply to learning at other levels of the personality including working with intuition. This kind of learning actually changes the energetic configurations of the personality. Once you learn to ride a bicycle, the skill is not something you can unlearn. Practice will refine your skill, but if you do not practice you will not forget the art of riding, and you will rapidly regain your skill if you try again.

Refusing to act if you feel unsure is still a decision. In medicine the student is taught that when in doubt, do nothing. This can be a good motto for a physician. But the advice is not for inaction or lack of decision. It might rather be called watchful waiting. This strategy may be needed at times to allow the physician to uncover the right timing for the therapeutic intervention. The disciple must learn that timing is everything. But you must also learn that you do not learn to walk by sitting on the floor because you are afraid to fall.

65. *Learn the art of unceasing worship. This is the essence of Bhakti Yoga.*

Keys for Contemplation

- The core practice at this stage of the path:
  Practising the Presence of God
  Meditation in action
- *Abhyasa* and *Vairagya* are the two wheels of the chariot of sadhana.
- **Strive for a state of intense, unceasing awareness of that Presence.**
- **The relationship with the Centre is not mediated; all convention, ritual and religion fall away.**
  No rules are needed on how to live life; one becomes internally rather than externally referenced.
- **This Path is only for the courageous.**
- **In this unceasing awareness, some are led by light and some by sound.**
- **The Centre answers with bliss and absorbs the awareness into It into absorption.**
- **The Centre is both point and expansion.**

You must learn the art of unceasing worship. Swami Rama used to talk about the chariot of *sadhana* with its two wheels of *abhyasa* (practice) and *vairagya* (detachment). The chariot needs two wheels to progress, with both turning together. At the point on the Path addressed by this book, these two practices simultaneously define the essence of one's spiritual *sadhana*.

In this sutra we deal with *abhyasa*. This is what would be called Practising the Presence of God in Christian literature. It might be called meditation in action in Yoga. Along with gaining detachment, this is the only basic practice there is at this stage. One is to hold that awareness of the Presence twenty-four hours a day without a gap until it becomes natural and spontaneous (*sahaja*), stable and unchangeable, as well as continuous.

The Bhakti Sutras (Prakash, 1998) address the importance of the art of unceasing worship.

> 35 "Spiritual devotion (ie awareness of the Centre of Consciousness) is developed by relinquishing objects and relinquishing attachments."

> 36 "By unceasing worship."

These two bhakti sutras delineate the importance of the two wheels of the chariot of *sadhana*: *vairagya* or nonattachment in sutra 35, and *abhyasa* or practice in bhakti sutra 36. These are referred to also in the *Yogasutras* (Aranya, 1981):

> "By practice and detachment these (ie mental activity) can be stopped."
> Yogasutras I.12

You will recall that "practice" in this context refers to the effort to acquire a tranquil state of mind devoid of mental activity (Yogasutras I.13). So what will be the content of such a mind? It will be the continuous and growing effulgence of the Centre of Consciousness. Speaking metaphorically, there are no ripples on the surface of the ocean of the mind to distort or obscure the view of its depths. Again from the Bhakti Sutras (Prakash, 1998):

> 49. "Renouncing even the scriptures, a complete, unceasing, intense longing for God is obtained."

The disciple must strive for a state of intense, unceasing awareness of that Presence within. The experience of spirit then becomes direct and spontaneous, providing immediate guidance and direction in the disciple's life. That relationship with spirit is not mediated through anyone or anything.

Swami Rama spoke of this many times. For detachment or nonattachment, he used the word "desirelessness". Until you are desireless you cannot have the peace of the Self, Whose first manifestation in the mind is the

Centre of Consciousness as we refer to it here. He spoke of meditation thus:

> "Whenever you have time, sit down quietly, compose yourself, and just start remembering that Centre deep down within you beyond the thinking process."

> "Desire is the very root of all miseries. You must become desireless and maintain the here and now [ie the awareness of the Centre] by constant awareness. Remember the Centre of Consciousness within you. Constant awareness is the most important thing, and it is possible for you to achieve. ... you must first become peaceful and tranquil"

> "You cannot experience anything of God if your mind remains agitated and dissipated by desires. You must first become calm, peaceful and tranquil. ... Just for a few seconds ask yourself not to have any desires. What will be the condition of your mind then? Immediately your mind will flow in an ocean of joy and bliss (ie be filled with the effulgence of the Centre). When you are able to lead your mind to the state of desirelessness, then it is considered to be real meditation. The purpose of meditation is to lead you to that higher state. ... if you attain that center within with the help of meditation, then you will have peace of mind."

> "You should learn to play your part while having constant awareness of the Reality that is within you. You should allow all the desires to be swallowed up by the one desire for attaining the higher purpose of life. ... When the desire to know God is strengthened, it swallows all other desires. Finally this desire is fulfilled by attaining a height beyond itself called desirelessness."
>
> Swami Rama, 1999b, p28

These few quotations show the interplay between detachment and practice of the Centre of Consciousness.

As the inner guidance unfolds all convention, ritual and religion fall away. The disciple needs no external rules on how to live life. He or she becomes internally rather than externally referenced, and the expression of the *yamas* and the *niyamas* in behaviour now becomes natural. This development may upset others since the disciple may stop behaving conventionally. He or she may be misunderstood and attacked by contemporaries. Look at what has been done over the centuries to persecute sages. The orthodox religious hierarchy may also feel threatened and disempowered by someone who no longer needs them as an intermediary to reach God.

A young man once approached Swami Rama to say that he wanted to renounce and go to the caves to work for enlightenment. Swamiji refused, and advised him instead to go into the world and to be successful. For Swamiji that usually meant getting a PhD and getting married! "First conquer the world," he said, "and then come back to me when you have something to renounce!" He then turned to the rest of the audience and said sternly, "This path is only for the courageous! This is a path of conquest!"

In this unceasing awareness of the Centre, some are led by light and some by sound. Some will hear the subtle sounds of the chakras in the right ear. This is the basis of nada yoga. Sometimes the sounds are quite loud and seem to fill whole body with their vibration.

As one offers that unceasing awareness to the Presence it soon flows as devotion and love. At times the Centre will seem to answer that unceasing worship with bliss that pours into the personality like a descending force, a force that can be quite hard on the personality and physical body to sustain for any length of time. It is important to prepare the personality to handle these higher energies by regular yoga practice. The Centre may seem to absorb one's awareness into It. There is no loss of awareness - just force, light, bliss, with or without the inner sounds, stillness, silence, and pure knowing and being. Sometimes the awareness is expanded and other times focussed to a point, representative of the symbol of a dot enclosed by a circle. It is interesting how the word "*samadhi*" is often translated as "absorption". In the *Yogasutras* (II.45), Patanjali is clear that the result of this one-pointed *Ishvara Pranidhana* is *samadhi*.

Bhakti yoga recognizes five *Bhavas* as follows (Prakash, 1998):

1. *Dasya Bhava*   Attitude of a servant
2. *Sakhya Bhava*   Attitude of a friend
3. *Vatsalya Bhava* Attitude of a parent
4. *Shanta Bhava*   Attitude of a philosopher
5. *Kanta Bhava*   Attitude of a spouse

These are five attitudes toward God that the disciple may assume. Traditionalists consider them to be hierarchical. But in practice they are simply mental attitudes used to cultivate spiritual devotion. The disciple assumes one of these attitudes to evolve a personal relationship with God. The particular attitude selected will reflect an individual's temperament so that the vibratory level of the energy of the personality can harmonize with the particular Divine manifestation, in this case, the Centre of Consciousness. At times the Centre presents Itself in a very impersonal fashion. At other times one experiences a

128 Sutras of the Inner Teacher

distinctive personal relationship with the Inner Teacher. Both manifestations go on together depending on the needs of the situation. But paradoxically it is actually the Divine who plays the role of both worshipper and worshipped. In the Ramayana, Hanuman says, "From the viewpoint of the body, I am Thy servant; from the viewpoint of the ego, I am a portion of Thee; from the viewpoint of the Self, I am Thyself." (Prakash, 1998).

66. *Learn never to take the Inner Teacher for granted. Learn to take the Inner Teacher for granted!*

Keys to Contemplation

- **The Bhagavad Gita records the dialogue between Arjuna (the qualified disciple) and Krishna (the Guru and Inner Teacher) in the context of the battlefield of life.**
- **The Presence always evokes feelings of respect, gratitude, praise, love and reverence.**
- **The Presence is nearer than near, dearer than dear, your own true Self.**
- **Not to follow your Spirit without hesitation to the best of your ability is to show disrespect.**

At the subtle level, the important text on Karma Yoga called the Bhagavad Gita (Swami Rama, 1985) records the dialogue between Arjuna, the qualified disciple, and Krishna, the Inner Guru or Inner Teacher - in this case the Centre of Consciousness. The dialogue takes place in the context of the battlefield of life.

> 41 "Thinking you my friend, what ever I said impetuously ... not knowing of this glory of yours, inadvertently as well as out of affection,
>
> 42 As I have been disrespectful out of jest in occasions of sport, sleep, or dining, alone or in the presence of others, O Infallible One, I beg You, a who are immeasurable, to forgive me."
> Bhagavad Gita XI

This quotation points to an important aspect of the relationship between the disciple and the Centre. On the one hand the disciple must learn never to take the Inner Teacher for granted. The effect that the Centre of Consciousness, the Presence, has on the disciple is to invoke always feelings of respect, gratitude, praise, love, and reverence. In this sense the disciple never takes It for granted.

But in a different sense the disciple learns always to take the Presence for granted! This paradox arises because the Presence is nearer than near because it is an expression of one's own true Self, and hence dearer than dear. As the trust and faith in the relationship grows it becomes so much a part of the disciple's experience that the guidance can always be assumed and counted on. However, the disciple will learn that the way in which the teaching occurs and the guidance comes may not meet the disciple's personal expectations. The guidance will always exceed those expectations in support of the disciple's best interests. Indeed, not to follow your Spirit without hesitation to the best of your ability is to show disrespect.

67. *Working with the Centre of Consciousness is practical.*

Keys to Contemplation

- **Experience your true attributes.**
- **Access the unconscious to identify and correct personal and social beliefs.**
    * **The role of kinesiology**
- **Guidance about the universe.**
- **Guidance about the body and health.**
- **Access the wisdom of the Tradition.**
- **Guidance about relationships.**
- **Guidance about right action.**

This sutra refers to the wisdom aspect of the Centre of Consciousness, its functioning as the Inner Teacher. The devotional nature of the Centre has been described above in sutra 65, and is the basis of Bhakti Yoga. The wisdom aspect becomes the basis of Jnana Yoga at this stage of the Path.

You will learn gradually to experience your true attributes. These are attributes of the Self, the soul. They include qualities such as love, light, bliss and joy, intelligence, Presence, peace, infinite energy, creativity, and abundance. You will learn of the law of allowing and how to become nonjudgmental. Quite simply, you are made in the image of your Creator and share Its attributes. It is one thing to know this intellectually, but quite another to begin to experience it as a personal reality. Own your own power.

You will learn how to access and work with the unconscious mind so that you can begin to live deliberately rather than by habit and default. You learn to identify and to correct both personal and societal belief systems that produce fear and that block the ability to manifest and to act effectively. This is done initially by establishing "Yes/No" signals to verify the correctness of the information received. You learn to distinguish intuitive from subconscious transmissions discovering how to translate the information contained in subtle vibrating mental fields into thoughts and language. A knowledge of applied kinesiology can be very useful here (Gallo, 1999; Thie, 1996). Communication with parts of the personality in Neuro-Linguistic Programming is another useful process (sutra 49) (Cameron-Bandler, 1985; O'Connor and Seymour, 1990; James and Woodsmall, 1988). Mind-body communication using ideodynamic signalling is also helpful (Rossi and Cheek, 1988).

You can access truths about the universe, or creative inspiration in the arts if you are a scientist or an artist.

You will learn to love yourself, including your physical body. You will learn to communicate with its parts by way of signals from the unconscious mind that controls the psychoneuroimmune system underlying host resistance. One learns that ultimately illness is a miscreation originating in the mind. Illnesses and symptoms have functional attributes and qualities of decisions at the mental level. They are adaptations that perform a useful function for the body at a time of crisis. How do you know when you are healthy? The concept of health is not useful when defined as the absence of disease. Health prevention is an ill-formed outcome since it focuses on what is not wanted rather than on what is wanted. Learn to sense the vibratory signal, the feel of perfect health, and how to use it to assist healing.

One can learn to assess the wisdom of an ascended master to interpret written texts, for example. The following quotation gives a clue as to how this is possible.

> "The Holy Ones are an Intelligence within your intellect.
> Give your profoundest contemplation to this."
> Jelaleddin Rumi

This quotation refers to the holographic nature of the universe. The wisdom of the macrocosm is fully contained within the microcosm of the personality. An example is a body cell. Each cell has a full complement of DNA that codes for the whole organism. It also has the information to direct the differentiation, development and expression of any individual cell within the organism. A particular cell grows and develops by suppressing the expression of any information not necessary to define its particular type or differentiated state. There is a metaphor here for the personality. If the individual is a kind of spiritual cell within the body of the universe, the wisdom of the Centre of Consciousness would be analogous to the DNA, with all individuals having access to that same total informational potential. A particular personality is a differentiation or particular manifestation or expression of that infinite intelligence into the time, space and causation of the physical universe. In other words, channelling the wisdom of a master is not about connecting with some entity "out there", somewhere, in some subtle dimension. It is about contacting that holographic representation within the infinite intelligence of the Centre of Consciousness present in all of us. Give your profoundest contemplation to the possibilities of this.

You can also receive guidance about relationships and about people within those relationships. Guidance is also available about the situations of everyday affairs.

You can receive guidance about the nature of right action in any situation. You learn to sense the right action to be taken in any situation regardless of what you or others may want personally. With this comes guidance on life missions, visions, and goals. There is also guidance on how to behave ethically in any situation.

Note that in all of this, moral behaviour is simply assumed. Note also that these are not *siddhis* or powers. In essence you can know anything that you need to know. You just have to ask and be able to receive and translate the transmission through intuition. But the frivolous and the curious bring no response. The guidance is on a "need to know" basis. You have to ask. And you have to respect the information you receive by acting on it.

Concluding Remarks on the Curriculum

How is this process of "channelling" the Centre of Consciousness to be done? Here is the essence of it.

WORKING WITH THE CENTRE OF CONSCIOUSNESS

- **Act "as if" the Centre is sufficiently open and accessible at least to some degree.**
- **Attune with the Centre by meditation for 10 minutes.**
- **"Ask" the question.**
- **"Translate" the response.**
- **Check its veracity with the Yes/No signal you have previously established until you are skilled enough not to need this.**
- **Write the response in a journal.**
- **Act as appropriate on the guidance received.**
- **This is a skill: practice, practice, practice!**

When the awareness of the Centre becomes stable the process becomes an ongoing "dialogue" without formalities of techniques.

These few sutras highlight a little of the curriculum for the new disciple. One might call it "Working with the Centre of Consciousness 101". We began this section with excerpts from the little manual, *Light on the Path*, and we conclude with some additional comments from that text on this initial curriculum.

> "II,14 Having obtained the use of the inner senses, having conquered the desires of the outer senses, having conquered the desires of the individual soul, and having obtained knowledge, prepare now, O disciple, to enter upon the way in reality. The path is found: make yourself ready to tread it.
>
> 15 Inquire of the earth, the air, and the water, of the secrets they hold for you. The development of your inner senses will enable you to do this.
>
> 16 Inquire of the holy ones of the earth of the secrets they hold for you. The conquering of the desires of the outer senses will give you the right to do this.
>
> 17 Inquire of the inmost, the one, of its final secret, which it holds for you

through the ages.

> The great and difficult victory, the conquering of the desires of the individual soul, is a work of ages; therefore expect not to obtain each reward until ages of experience have been accumulated. When the time on learning this seventeenth rule is reached, man is on the threshold of becoming more than man."
>
> Collins, 1976, pp 13 - 14

IV THE ATTUNEMENT

Attaining Spiritual Devotion

68. *Attainment of the Centre of Consciousness is threefold.*

We now reach to the core, the essence of what we choose to call *samahita yoga*, the Yoga of the Centre of Consciousness. This and the next two sutras show that its attainment is threefold. We have reviewed the role of *abyhasa*, practice, and *vairagya*, detachment, using the metaphor of the two wheels of the chariot of *sadhana* (sutra 65). The third component, of course, is the Centre itself. Through practice of unceasing awareness and remembrance there is a continual invoking of the Presence with Its response of love, bliss and wisdom. By detachment the *sadhaka* purifies the mind progressively by releasing attachments and aversions (*raga* and *dvesha*) that provide the emotional drive which fills the mind with continual, compulsive thoughts and desires. This combination of practice and detachment leads eventually to a still, stable and peaceful mind field into which the effulgence of the Centre flows naturally.

> "Know the Atman to be the master of the chariot; the body, the chariot; the buddhi, the charioteer; and the mind, the reins."
> Kathopanishad I.iii.3

In this quotation the word "Atman" refers to the *jiva*, the living being and aspect of pure consciousness that appears through *maya* as the embodied soul subject to space, time and causation - the experiencer of the results of action. The body is compared to a chariot that is moved here and there by the sense organs which are compared to horses.

The word *buddhi* denotes the discriminative faculty, the intellect, which has the power of discrimination and determination. An individual depends mainly for his or her action upon the *buddhi*, which determines what he or she should be doing and what he or she should refrain from doing. Through the

134 Sutras of the Inner Teacher

mind the *buddhi* directs the senses to their respective objects just as a charioteer guides the horses along the right path by means of reins.

If the intellect relates to an uncontrolled mind that is always distracted it loses discrimination. Then the senses become uncontrolled like the vicious horses of a charioteer. But if the intellect relates to a mind that is restrained and possesses discrimination, then the senses come under control like the good horses of a charioteer. The disciple who has discrimination for his charioteer always holds the reins of mind firmly, and reaches the end of the road where he obtains an uninterrupted vision of all-pervading consciousness. Intuitive wisdom from the Centre of Consciousness reflected into the inner face of *buddhi*, the intellect, provides it with unerring discrimination.

A similar metaphor in the Bhagavad Gita, often presented as an illustration, shows the qualified disciple Arjuna steering his chariot in the battlefield of life with the guidance of Krishna (the Inner Teacher) who rides with him.

69. One is purification through detachment.

70. One is unceasing worship with a still, one-pointed mind.

71. Most important is the grace of God through the blessing of a great soul.

So if this is some of the beginning curriculum, How, besides detachment (purification) and unceasing worship (a still, one pointed mind), is spiritual devotion to the Centre of Consciousness (the Inner Teacher) to be attained?

Narada's Bhakti Sutras put it nicely (Prakash, 1998):

38. "But primarily from the mere grace of God via the blessing of a great soul.

39. But the companionship of a great soul is difficult to obtain. It is unfathomable, and it is infallible."

If you were not meant to see Swami Rama there was no way that you could get to him. We recall an episode with a Canadian colleague who visited our rural outreach program as it was being developed from the campus of the Himalayan Institute Hospital Trust near Rishikesh in foothills of the Himalayas in India. He had heard a great deal about Swamiji and very much wished to meet him. Many attempts were set up for a meeting which did not materialize.

One hot and sunny afternoon he went to see the small school on the campus and just as he disappeared inside the door, Swamiji drove up in his jeep. We thought that at last a meeting would be possible since our friend would finish his tour very quickly. The time passed as we conversed with Swamiji but our friend did not appear. Our conversation finished and Swamiji climbed back into his jeep. Just as he drove away our friend appeared. Even down to a split second timing that meeting was not to take place. On the other hand, if you are ready to meet your master you cannot avoid that meeting, even if you bump into him in the lineup at the airport.

> 40. "Only by God's grace is their companionship even obtained.
>
> 41. Because there is no difference between the grace of God and those great souls arising from that grace,
>
> 42. Cultivate grace alone; cultivate grace alone."
> (Prakash, 1998)

And that grace includes not only the *darshan* and guidance of the guru, but also higher initiation in the form of *shaktipat*. Paramahamsa Yogananda used to say that twenty-five percent was your own effort; twenty-five percent was the Guru's effort, and fifty percent was the grace of God.

> "It is said that the winds of grace are always blowing. But to catch them you must raise your sail!"
> Ramakrishna

In short, the guidance of a competent, enlightened Guru is essential. In the Himalayan Tradition such a being is defined by the ability to give higher spiritual initiations, such as *shaktipat*. The guidance is usually in the form of a physical master, and may be as short as a single meeting with only a word or two exchanged, or it may be for a long period of service and training, depending on the disciple's need. Occasionally the guidance comes in other ways, such as a dream, but such events are rare and easily misinterpreted. When the student is ready, the master will appear.

72. *Spiritual devotion is also Ishvara Pranidhana*

Keys for Contemplation

- Ishvara (the Lord) is an impersonal, transcendental Self that governs the cosmos and individuated beings.
- The first and root Guru of all spiritual philosophy and Yoga.
- Both an impersonal spiritual energy and a personal Presence.
- Called "the spirit of guidance" by the Sufis.
    - The "Holy Ghost" in Christianity
    - The "Voice for God" in the *Course in Miracles*
- The first experience is personal.
    - * The ego lives in personal, subject-object consciousness.
    - * Enlightened men and women are manifestations of Ishvara.
- Unceasing worship of the Centre of Consciousness is *Ishvara Pranidhana*.
- *Hiranyagarbha*, the Golden Womb, is the Teaching Spirit of the universe.

This discussion now raises the question of *Ishvara* and *Ishvara Pranidhana* as set forth in Patanjali's *Yogasutras* (Aranya, 1981).

23. "From special devotion to Isvara also (concentration becomes imminent).

24. Ishvara is a particular Purusha unaffected by affliction, deed, result of action or latent impressions thereof.

25. In Him the seed of omniscience has reached its utmost development which cannot be exceeded.

26. (He is) The teacher of former teachers because with Him there is no limitation by time (to his omnipotence).

27. The sacred word designating Him is Pranava or the mystic syllable OM.

28 (Yogins) Repeat it and contemplate upon its meaning.

29. From that comes realization of the individual self and the obstacles are resolved.
Yogasutras I

45. From devotion to God (Ishvara Pranidhana), samadhi is attained.
Yogasutras II

This reference to *Ishvara*, the Lord, is found in the yogic writings as early as the *Brihad-Aranyaka Upanishad*, portions of which may date back to 1500 BC, as well as in many of the Vedanta-influenced schools. *Ishvara* is often referred to in an impersonal sense as a transcendental Self that governs the cosmos and individuated beings.

It is Patanjali in the *Yogasutras* who first makes reference to *Ishvara* in a devotional sense. He refers to *Ishvara* as the first guru, the first teacher of spiritual philosophy and Yoga. *Ishvara* is the root guru of all yogic teachings.

73. The experience of Ishvara is both personal and transpersonal.

Ishvara can be experienced as a both an impersonal spiritual energy, and as a personal Presence that can be realized by the yogi. The reader might recall Swami Rama's mission referred to earlier: "My job is to introduce you to the Teacher within." When we asked Swamiji what this internal Presence was, he replied quite simply, "It is the Lord." Later one of us became confused as to the difference between internal worship of the guru and the Presence. A clear and compelling internal experience was given by the Master to show that the two were one and the same (sutra 39).

The Sufis say that when the universe of illusion first became manifest, the *sat-cit-ananda* assumed a role as "the spirit of guidance." The Sufis consider this to be God in the role of divine teacher to those in bondage to illusion. In Christianity the analogous concept is the Holy Ghost, the Teaching Spirit of the universe (Arya, 1979). It is called the Voice for God in the *Course in Miracles* (1975).

If *Ishvara* is a transcendental spiritual consciousness then how can It be experienced also in a personal sense? Since the individual ego lives in subject-object consciousness, its experiences of God are also very personal in the same way that the ego experiences itself as the self-reflexive aspect of personal consciousness (Varela, Thompson and Rosch, 1991). Later when the soul transcends yogic identity then the transcendental nature of *Ishvara* will also be realized.

74. Enlightened Masters are manifestations of Ishvara.

This spirit of guidance first becomes manifest through enlightened human beings. Enlightened men and women are manifestations of *Ishvara*. The personal relationship established with a master becomes the doorway to the transpersonal and transcendent experience of spiritual consciousness. "I am the way, the truth, and the life: no man cometh unto the Father, but by me." (St. John 14:6).

The unceasing worship of the Centre of Consciousness means the unceasing worship of *Ishvara*. It is the basis of Bhakti Yoga (sutra 65). As though drawn by the spiritual magnet of that devotion Ishvara fills the empty vacuum of egolessness thus created by the yogi with the energy of spiritual guidance.

75. Hiranyagarbha alone is the teacher of yoga.

Hiranyagarbha, the Golden Womb, is another designation for the Inner Teacher.

> "Hiranyagarbha alone is the teacher of Yoga, and no other."
> Brhad-yogi-yajnavalkya-smrti XII.5

For yogis there is no individual person who is a teacher, a master, or a guru. At no time did Swami Rama refer to himself as such - only as a messenger come to introduce us to the Teacher within. The Golden Womb alone is the guru (Arya, 1986, p69). When one is freed from individual identification as a separate ego then all the knowledge of the Golden Womb flows into the mind effortlessly and naturally through an awakened intuition. In meditation such a one does not know himself or herself as separate from the Golden Womb. Thus all revelation is grace that flows from the Golden Womb into minds in meditation. When the master initiates a disciple into Its mysteries the disciple experiences a golden luminosity within and the dawning of intuitive knowledge.

Although *Ishvara* is usually translated by the word "God", this is meant not as a person but as a superior spiritual consciousness that is so pure that it is completely free of any relationship with karma and its effects (Swami Satyananda Saraswati, 1989, p83). Different commentators explain this sutra in different ways. Some say that it means that *samadhi* is obtained by self-surrender to God. Others say that *samadhi* is obtained by fixing the mind on the Lord. Still others say that it is the awareness which is to be placed in God. The word "*pranidhana*" has the meaning of "placing completely, absolutely, thoroughly". Thus *Ishvara pranidhana* means that the disciple completely places his or her awareness, the mind, the thought and consciousness into *Ishvara*.

Transpersonal Visioning: The Art of Loving Wisdom in Action

Keys to Contemplation
Creating a Spiritual Vision
(Next Life Planning)

- The power of paradigms and the law of cause and effect.
- Shift your paradigms.
- Under the guidance from the Centre create the highest vision you can about who you truly are.
- You can only create what you can imagine.
- Test every thought, word and action against this vision. Does it serve me?
- Recreate yourself in increments; step-by-step you will reach the summit.

We conclude here with a more modern version of how to think about the Centre of Consciousness in action (Alarius and Polaria, 1990). It will provide the reader with a very different view of the process, perhaps with a new millennial perspective.

Although the Truth is but One, it can be expressed in many ways depending on the properties of its particular point of expression in time, space and causation. A metaphor may be helpful here. White light is broken into its constituent colours by a refracting prism. That part of the prism that transmits the colour red will be understood by, will resonate intellectually with, those who can receive and understand the meaning of redness. Similarly for each of the other spectral colours. Each colour is a part of the whole of white light, but not its completeness. A summation of all the colours would give the completeness of white light. The more colours one could accept, the closer one would understand the completeness that is whiteness. Similarly the more different ways that one can hear the Truth expressed the deeper becomes one's understanding. Expressions of the Truth that are very different from and that challenge one's current understanding can be especially valuable in helping a student integrate a much deeper understanding. Synthesizing the apparent dissonance of a very different point of view with one's own understanding can lead to a greater appreciation of the common themes that underlie the two.

Up to this point we have shown how this yoga of the Centre of Consciousness is integral, providing a synthesis of the yogas of life with the yogas of discipline. Of the former we have dealt with both Bhakti and Jnana Yogas to this point. Now we will show how Karma Yoga is integrated. The key is to understand that the laws of karma as the laws of cause and effect are really the laws of creativity in the sense of manifestation. Karma Yoga, then, becomes the yoga of creativity, of divine manifestation in the world.

76. *Understand the creative power of paradigms.*

In the metaphor above of the refraction of white light into its constituent colours by a crystal, for what function is the crystal the analogy? For this, one needs a practical working model of mind, and to understand how the mind constructs our moment to moment experience by creating models of reality. All this has been presented above in sutras 21 and 22 and should be reviewed here. One has not to look far to see the profound practical implications of cognitive paradigms.

But we have referred in this sutra to the <u>creative</u> power of paradigms. In thinking about Karma Yoga there are three key ingredients. The first is the Centre of Consciousness because true Karma Yoga is action flowing with awareness from the Centre of Consciousness. The second is one's model of the world. One's belief systems determine one's boundaries of self-identity as well as what one believes is real and therefore what one believes is possible. You are effectively what you believe and that is part of your bondage. That mental structure constructed from life experience by the intellect filters the transmission of intent from Spirit, diluting its force and distorting its thrust to varying degree. The resulting desire determines the thoughts, words and deeds that constitute action in the world and that generate the resulting karmic feedback through cause and effect. The third component then involves the process of manifestation itself, which we will now discuss.

77. *To radically change your life the most powerful thing you can do is to change your models of reality.*

If you accept the importance of belief systems, of models of the world then you will realize their importance in creating your experience of reality. Thus it follows that the most powerful thing you can do to change your experience of reality, your existence, is to be able to change your models of the world. Of the three components of Karma Yoga mentioned above, being able to shift paradigms is the weakest link. The ability to change your beliefs, attitudes and values remains the key skill in this three-part sequence.

When a mental paradigm changes, it does so in a characteristic pattern. Much like a system in general systems theory, the force for change provided by external input of experience and information builds against the internal homeostatic resistance inherent in the models to reach a threshold. Then a sudden, irreversible expansion of insight called a paradigm shift occurs, which the individual may experience as an "aha" reaction. The mental paradigm or model of the world has now been irreversibly changed so that this person no longer reacts to the situation in the same way. The new world view includes, but is a major expansion of the old one, and hence introduces greater flexibility and choices for more effective coping behaviours.

THE PARADIGM SHIFT
- The current paradigm (status quo) is the grand answer for all.
- Troublesome anomalies build to a point of crisis.
- A new and heretical insight arises.
- The new contains the old as a special case.
- The new is greeted with hostility and indifference.
- To accept the new, one must let go of the old.
- The new comes as a sudden illumination.

Adapted from Kuhn, 1962

The best model for this paradigm shift comes surprisingly from Thomas Kuhn's work in the philosophy of science (Kuhn, 1962). He described the paradigm shift in his book, *The Structure of Scientific Revolutions*. The concept is easier to grasp when it is presented in the format of belief change in science as he originally described it.

"A paradigm is a framework of thought for understanding and explaining certain areas of reality. When a paradigm shifts, a distinctly new way of thinking about old problems emerges.

The paradigm shift in physics is usually given as the most potent example. At the turn of the century Isaac Newton's paradigm of a predictable mechanical universe held sway. A grand answer for the whole natural scheme was in sight with only a few troubling bits and pieces here and there that refused to fit and needed tidying up. But as the anomalous observations piled up to a point of crisis a new principle, a new and heretical insight arose which resolved the apparent contradictions. Quantum mechanics and the special theory of relativity became the new paradigm to supercede Newtonian mechanics. Our view of nature shifted from a clockwork paradigm of absolute predictability to an uncertainty paradigm which was relative. The new perspective contained the old paradigm as a special case. Given its wider scope and power, one would have expected the new paradigm to have prevailed quickly. Kuhn points out that this almost never happens. The new paradigm cannot be accepted unless one lets go of the old, and the new comes as a sudden illumination rather than as a gradual 'figuring out'.

>Thus new paradigms are almost always received with hostility at worst and indifference at best. Their discoverers in history have been attacked as heretics (Copernicus, Galileo, Pasteur, Mesmer). Kuhn asserts that established scientists are often not converted because of the demanding change that the new perspective requires. Their attachment to the old way of thinking is habituated if not emotional, and they may finish their careers with their faith unshaken. Even when confronted with overwhelming data for the new paradigm they may continue to stick stubbornly with the familiar, "My mind's made up, don't confuse me with facts!"
>
> Jerry, 1985

This paradigm shift describes the process of learning from experience, which involves a change in beliefs. This is not learning based on the gathering of information, but the acquisition of real wisdom.

Whether a particular situation, for example mountain climbing, is experienced as an exciting challenge, a neutral event or a stressful threat is a matter of individual perception. Host resistance responds in kind, for behaviour is truly a biologic response modifier. This also highlights a point of control. The trick is not necessarily trying to change the external situation (although that may be appropriate in some cases), but rather one's subjective experience of it. This is the great blessing of nonattachment bestowed by the meditative tradition.

78. *Generate a life vision of extraordinary beingness under the guidance of the Centre of Consciousness.*

Use the creative power of mental paradigms to generate deliberately a vision for one's life under the guidance of the Centre of Consciousness. It should be a vision of extraordinary beingness, a practical philosophy of life that can be used as a blueprint for action.

There are many popular works that can be consulted about the process of life planning. The whole field of strategic planning in management addresses this requirement for an organization so that it may conduct its business in focussed and efficient way. Strategic planning is really the same process we are talking about here applied to groups. It is a methodology for group creating and manifesting. But surprisingly few of us realize that we can use the same process not only to plan, but also to create our own life experience (9).

You must accept that you alone are the architect of your life; you create your own destiny. Be prepared to take the necessary responsibility to live consciously and to create your life with awareness. Unfortunately most of us are unable to do this, much less realize that such a thing is even possible.

These days we hear much about rights and freedoms. But what we really need is a charter of responsibilities! For rights and freedoms flow from conscious and responsible living and not the reverse. As conscious creators of our destinies, life owes us nothing; we are free to create anything we want.

> You are what your deepest driving desire is.
> As your deepest driving desire is, so is your will.
> As your will is, so is your deed.
> And as your deed is, so is your destiny.
> Upanishads

79. Perform actions established in yoga.

Yogasthah kuru karmani (Bhagavad Gita II.48): established in yoga, perform actions. Krishna as the Inner Teacher enlightens the qualified disciple, Arjuna, as to the true nature of Karma Yoga, of selfless action, "First establish yourself in Me," he says, "and then take up a line of service." This is certainly an appropriate motto for a life lived in Spirit. Here, of course, the word "yoga" means union with the Centre of Consciousness. Perform action in conscious union with that Centre. Karma Yoga is action flowing from the Centre of Consciousness. To do this you need to distinguish background versus foreground creating.

All pictures of reality can be considered to have both a foreground and a background (Alarius, 1991). Most planning processes address only the foreground with the background assumed to be a given. People do not realize they could create a new background. Foreground reality is always a logical extension of the structure of one's background reality.

To create a powerful vision for personal change, you create a new background from which the foreground will emerge spontaneously. The generality of the mission creates the background or context. The vision can be used to co-create a whole new background reality for yourself in which you live as an element in the foreground with a fuller expression of your potential. From new visions emerge new realities.

Your personal vision should have no attachment to anything particular in the world of form such as people, places, things, ideas or concepts. Your emotions will try to form these attachments as you go, limiting the possibilities of the vision by demanding certain boundaries and constraints. This is asking Spirit to co-create a magnificent vision with you, but to do it "my way". Unfortunately "my way" will yield a significantly lesser result. Be detached about the details and about how it will all unfold. Trust deeply in the appropriateness of the synchronicities that will manifest as, metaphorically speaking, the universe "rearranges itself" to accommodate your desired vision (Alarius and Polaria, 1990).

Your basic identity is the background-you as a core spiritual being. The foreground-you will be the idiosyncrasies of your physical/emotional/mental personality that constitute the vehicle for your physical expression in the world as well as the role you play in life. Since your vision aims at co-creating yourself as a master of divine expression - a karma yogi- this gives you a transpersonal background reality from which you can play any role that expresses this in the foreground, be it teacher, healer, guide or whatever. You may play several of these roles during a lifetime, each tied to developing mastery of divine expression from the Centre. Your real identity is transpersonal; the others are just roles that you play. Do not confuse the two. Thus foreground is your day to day, moment to moment life. Let your vision be focussed on choosing the background against which your life will be played.

The background reality always determines what the foreground reality will be like. Most of us just accept the background reality as a given, and never question it. We never imagine that we could change it. We do the best we can in the foreground reality to adapt. We try to manipulate ourselves in the foreground without changing the background. Instead of allowing the universal creative processes to work for us, we think only of trying to do it all ourselves. The result is continual frustration with our attempts to be all of whom we could be, because we do not have the big picture, a background reality that is big enough to accommodate all of our creating.

Using a metaphor, we spend all of our efforts painting a bird in our picture, trying to make it fit in to the forest background even though it is a sea gull. Try as we might the foreground image of this kind of bird does not adapt properly to the forest background. It does not occur to us that our frustration could be solved by recreating the background reality as a seascape. You are not big enough to unfold the grandest vision of who and what you are by simply manipulating the foreground, the daily issues of life, through your own personal action. Let the universe do it and then participate wholeheartedly, engaging in the vision as it unfolds, and doing your part when it comes.

What do we mean by "the universe" in this metaphor? The manifested universe is an infinitely complex system of energies permeated and sustained by consciousness. Like any system, a change induced by one part evokes an adaptive response by the whole as a restructuring or reorganizing of the system. Each of us is a part of that larger whole, and our actions also induce a response from the energetic whole that we experience most prominently as synchronicity. Through what some have called the law of attraction (Hicks and Hicks, 1988; 1991), the response always results in an experienced reality that reflects what is wanted.

The process of manifestation involves using visioning to activate that adaptive energetic response and then to be able to recognize and engage the synchronicities as they unfold. What is accomplished through personal action, doing it yourself, is a very small part of the process when one tries to manifest a large vision. This response from the universal energy is called many things: Shakti and Divine Mother are two terms used in yoga.

Swami Rama was a master at grand manifestation. He referred to this process continually in terms of the love and grace of Divine Mother. He perceived that She showered him with support and resources without his having to make it happen, force it to happen in the way we typically think that things evolve. Simply put, if you are having to struggle to get things to happen around you then you have not understood this process. Here we use the metaphorical idea of the universe " rearranging itself to accommodate our pictures of reality" that we generate through the visioning process (Alarius and Polaria, 1990).

This process is iterative. One systematically builds and rebuilds one's vision over and over. As soon as all that one can imagine has manifested, then it is time to create another and even bigger vision. One always stretches the limit of what one can envision. With each manifestation comes the ability to conceive of even further possibilities for creating an even larger vision. Each vision will have all of the same twelve background elements, but will grow bigger in an ongoing process (10).

80. You can only create what you can imagine.

Imagination plays an important role in this creative process. In the West we often downgrade the value of imagination. The comments, "It's only imaginary" or "It's all in your imagination," stress our collective belief in the unreality of the faculty of imagination as something best left to the entertainment of bored children on a rainy day.

But in actual fact it is the engine of creativity. Nothing was ever manifested on this planet by human effort without first existing as an idea in someone's mind. In that sense all creations are initiated in the mind. The realm of ideas and the process of using them creatively is the essence of visioning. Imagination is the foundation of creativity in general. It is the art of exploring the possible. So in this sense one can only create what one can imagine, and acquiring skills in visualizing and lateral thinking is a very good investment of time and effort.

But there is a built-in limitation of imagination. It can only rearrange, however creatively, mental content from memory based on past experience and learning. Simply put, if something is unimaginable for you then it cannot be manifested.

But the universal synchronicities inherent in the process of manifestation in response to a vision usually expand possibilities beyond what is initially imagined in the guiding vision. Hence it is important not to limit the vision by laying down rigid requirements about how it is to manifest. Be very clear and allowing about what is wanted and leave the details as much as possible to Spirit. As the synchronicities unfold they will delight you with their creative originality, opening doors and presenting new possibilities if you are alert and focussed enough to recognize them. Synchronicity favours the prepared mind. Things turn out much better than if you had planned the details yourself. You can have no better co-creative partner than Spirit working with the universal forces of the Divine Mother for producing best results! With experience the disciple develops trust in the process and skill in working with it. One learns the real meaning of "Yoga is skill in action.".

As these new possibilities unfold you can expand what can be imagined, what can be envisioned as the next steps. Once the current vision is manifested you move on to the next step, using these expanded possibilities for visioning that could not have been conceived of in the first round. The process becomes an expanding and evolving one.

81. Recreate yourself under the guidance of Spirit in increments until your life vision of extraordinary beingness is fully manifested.

The process described in the last sutra now leads to an incremental process of visioning and manifestation that progressively expands and unfolds the personality, eventually to the fullness of enlightenment. The process is co-creative with Spirit, with the Centre of Consciousness, which is another way of saying that personal development occurs under the ongoing and intimate guidance of the Inner Teacher working through everyday life experience.

More than being an unfoldment, it is as much a continual and incremental re-creation of the personality under the guidance of Spirit until the instrument is capable of the full expression of the Centre of Consciousness into matter. In other words, the creation of an enlightened master. At the level of intent the process is fully aware and conscious as an ongoing interaction with the Inner Teacher at every level of life from the mundane to the holy.

Keys to Contemplation

Spiritual visioning

Your vision will include three shifts:
- Shift your identity.
- Shift your life context.
- Shift your way of measuring reality.

82. Transform your identity.

Keys to Contemplation

Spiritual Visioning
1. Transform Your Identity

- The political self (ego) has mastered limitation.
- Learn to live transpersonally by mastering divine expression.
- To master divine expression is to master Karma Yoga, for Karma Yoga is action flowing from the Centre of Consciousness.

The first of these key shifts is one involving self identity. When the consciousness is identified with *buddhi* the ego is born as the sense of limited personal self. Indeed the ego has been called the *political self*. One need only watch the behaviours of the characters in a soap opera or of politicians in debate on television to know what is meant by this term "political self". When expressing as the ego, consciousness becomes limited by the model of the world or the pictures of reality with which it has identified itself. While that process is necessary for consciousness to experience a physical reality, the blueprint of the model of the world also provides the boundaries of limitation. These boundaries represent the values, beliefs and cause-effects that constitute the content of one's model of the world. They create the meaning of one's sensory experience and the experience of what is considered to be reality. It is this experience of apparent reality that creates the boundary. In the modern psychology these beliefs and experiences of reality, including psychological boundaries, are intricately coded (and can be modified) in sensory submodalities of mental imagery (Andreas and Andreas, 1987).

Because of its sense of isolation as a small self, the ego feels alone and is effectively separated from Spirit; it has no direct experience or evidence that Spirit exists. Yet such a small self exhibits mastery! It has achieved mastery of limitation! If you read popular magazines and newspapers and watch television you have to be impressed with the intelligence, skill, artistry and cleverness with which limited human beings can mess up their lives and the lives of others! If this cleverness could be harnessed to the service of the planet and humanity, the world would be a very different place today. But this kind of altruism will not come to the human race until the Centre of Consciousness opens in awareness in each individual. Humanity will be changed from within, person by person.

Yet the science of Yoga tells us that one's true identity is not the political self. You are the Self, ever pure, ever wise, ever free - Consciousness. And the first inkling of your true nature as the Self comes with the beginning manifestation of the Centre of Consciousness within, the Inner Teacher.

A story is commonly told in the Tradition about a lion cub whose mother was killed by hunters. The cub was very young and was adopted by a flock of sheep. The cub grew to behave like a sheep, wandering with the herd, bleating loudly and eating grass. One day a fully grown lion was out hunting and came across the herd. It was astounded to see the young cub among the sheep, for by now it was almost fully grown, and was even more amazed to see it behave like a sheep. The lion took the cub aside but was unsuccessful in persuading it that it was truly a lion and not a sheep. The cub did not understand until the lion took it to a pool of water where it could see its reflection and recognize the truth of its existence as a lion. Once the cub was clear about its true identity it was able to roam the forest as a hunter filling the air with the sound of mighty roars as befitted a true lion.

The awareness of the Centre of Consciousness is a qualitatively, totally new experience in the disciple's inner world. He or she must now begin to live surrendered to, one with, absorbed in, and identified with that Centre, with Spirit, however the disciple can imagine it for now. You are That. The identity transformation or shift means to learn to live transpersonally, not as a master of limitation, but now as a master of divine expression. The latter phrase characterizes an enlightened human being. Swami Rama lived as a master of divine expression. A Karma Yogi is a master of divine expression: action (karma) done in a state of inner divine union (yoga). Karma Yoga is action flowing from the Centre of Consciousness through the personality as a surrendered instrument.

Paul Brunton, a jnana yogi and student of Ramana Maharshi, described what he called the "short path" (Brunton, 1988). It involves constantly reminding ourselves of our true nature. This is the identity shift described here. The practice "begins and ends with the goal itself" (Brunton, 1988).

> "The notion that we must wait and wait while we slowly progress out of enslavement into liberation, out of ignorance into knowledge, out of the present limitations into a future union with the Divine, is only true if we let it be so. But we need not. We can shift our identification from the ego to the Overself [Self] in our habitual thinking, in our daily reactions and attitudes, in our response to events and the world ... By incessantly remembering what we really are, here and now at this very moment, we set ourselves free. Why wait for what already is?"
> Brunton, 1988

The short path is a testimony to the philosophy and co-creative power of the faculty of imagination and the power of "as if." But Brunton warns us not to take up the short path until we have laid a solid foundation in the basics. "The danger of the Short Path, and of the 'As If' exercise, is to fall into deception of oneself, or even into charlatanic deception of others." (Brunton, 1988). You can delude both yourself and others.

> "Carl Jung would say that such individuals have made the fatal error of actually identifying with the archetype of the god-man, or mana-man as he called it - the idea of god incarnate. This brings about a powerful 'inflation' of the personality, so that the person seems to become bigger than life. From contact with the archetype, such people may gain considerable charisma, like a high static electrical charge picked up from contact with a generator. They may attract large numbers of followers at much risk to themselves and

everyone concerned."

Combs, 1995

In short, the identification is not transcendental and the awareness is still caught in the subtler levels of the mind.

This danger inherent in misunderstanding the significance of the identity shift cannot be overemphasized. This transformation of identity is not something forced or achieved by the ego using some kind of practice. The key to avoiding the trap is the presence in the mind of Spirit as the Centre of Consciousness or Inner Teacher. The process is one of surrender to the Presence through constant remembrance. It is the essence of personal humility and simplicity. The Inner Teacher is real, not something imaginary conjured up by the mind in an "as if" process (as useful as that can be in the beginning to start the process off). Worship of the reality of the Inner Teacher in surrender will lead gently and surely to the identity shift naturally and in right timing. The point here is that the belief system of the aspirant should be such as to support and not block (from religious conditioning) this transition in consciousness as it occurs. A mature identity shift is the first phase of enlightenment.

83. *Recreate your life context*

Keys to Contemplation

Spiritual Visioning
2. Recreate Your Life Context

- **Release the belief that you project on the universe, that you are a limited, struggling being trapped in either a karmic or an educational system from which you must struggle to earn or to learn your way out, for the universe will reflect your beliefs back to you as your experience.**
- **You are not here to escape from the planet. You are here to manifest your co-creative mastery of expression from the Centre of Consciousness with all of the other nearly six billion potential masters currently on the planet.**
- **Can there be any higher purpose for a life lived at the time of the planetary transition at the dawn of the new millennium?**

❁

This shift involves playing a different role in life as a result of the change to background creating described in sutra 79. Many of us have created a background that determines a karmic system in which as a student one must struggle to earn one's way off the planet. Others of us have created the context of an educational system in which the individual as a student must struggle to learn one's way off the planet. These are examples of background realities as described in sutra 79. In the karmic background, karmic misdemeanours created in present and past lives have to be worked through and cleared. In this context some even speak of destiny. On the other hand, life presents challenges and lessons to a student who must learn by mastering these in a background that determines an educational system. In other words, the events are neutral. The concepts of karma or life lessons are interpretations overlaid on to these neutral events. Whether you experience them as karma or as lessons depends on the belief systems inherent in your model of the world. Models of the world create your experience of reality. These background constructed realities are in themselves neither true nor false, but may or may not be useful as a map to take you on your journey. As maps their utility can free you, but as rigid belief systems of what is right or wrong they can bind you with chains as strong as the beliefs are held. The emotional value (i.e. what is experienced as important about these beliefs) invested in a model of the world is what creates the attachment and bondage. Hold your models lightly as guides, hypotheses, or maps - in other words with detachment, and then let their light lead you on the Path.

Make no mistake here. We are not at all implying that the universe is not real or that the laws of cause and effect do not exist. Rather we refer here to the process by which you build the beliefs and values which give the meaning that creates your experience of that reality. These interpretations of the meaning of what is real are what are relative to each individual. You can choose to change them to create a more useful experience of what is real.

To recreate your life context means to move away from either a karmic or educational system in which you as a student must struggle to earn or to learn your way out of here. In other words, as interpretations of reality, models of the world are relative - you can choose how you will map reality. Make choices that are useful. The issue is to move away from models of the world that create an experience of struggle. This statement will upset many deeply held beliefs. But either background is a belief system that you project on to the universe of processes. The role that you play as a student in either of these backgrounds is not who you really are, only who you imagine that you are. That is not to say that playing these roles at a certain point on the spiritual path is not useful.

❃

Playing these roles can be very helpful at certain points in development. But there comes time when role playing needs to be transcended. Both of these roles portray you as a limited struggling being. If that is what you believe you are, then that is what you experience. The universal co-creative process knows only the command "yes". Some people formulate this in what they call a "law of attraction". The universal process unfailingly gives you what you ask for as a match to your vibration (the net negative or positive vibratory frequency of the energy you experience as emotion) as determined by your model of the world or pictures of reality acting as a blueprint.

The implication of the identity shift or transformation is that you are not here to escape from the planet. You are here to wake up to your true identity as an enlightened being, as the Self, and then to attempt to manifest more and more of the spiritual mastery that is yours into this material dimension.

Every individual on the planet has the same potential. Clearly there is no higher purpose for your life as we enter the new millennium and perhaps face a planetary shift that has been prophesied by so many for so long.

In the business world one hears a lot about partnering. However one may define that, the identity shift in a co-creative relationship means to partner with God as expressed through the Centre of Consciousness in the act of manifestation (Carroll, 1998). Partnering is commonly thought of as occurring between equals, each of whom brings something unique to the partnership. In the West we are not accustomed to this kind of relationship with God. Review again the various relationships in the Bhakti Tradition between the devotee and God in sutra 65. Review the relationship between Arjuna and Krishna in the Bhagavad Gita. These are co-creative partnerships as we mean them here. Just as the worker is considered to be worthy of his hire, so is the sincere disciple. Perhaps a metaphor from management could be useful here. In a co-creative partnership with the Centre of Consciousness, the Centre acts as the inspiration and architect for action, while the ego acts as project manager for the process of manifestation. Both are essential functions for the process of divine manifestation called Karma Yoga.

In a karmic system there is an overlay of good and bad implied as a judgment to actions. The laws of karma are simply the laws of cause and effect, the laws of manifestation. Whether they are considered good or bad is a judgment projected by the individual. Even the concept of destiny has an element of judgment. If I fall from tree and break my leg, was that my destiny? Was I being punished for past sin? Was I reaping the consequences of negative past action? Or perhaps I could escape responsibility for my actions by saying that my fall was because of bad karma, or by blaming the injury on bad luck. But in a lawful universe of cause and effect the concept of chance makes no sense. Scientists have evolved a mathematics of probability to help them recognize causal relationships. Excluding the micro-universe of quantum physics, in everyday life one cannot have one's cake and eat it too. Einstein noted that God does not play with dice. The idea of bad luck is more a social excuse and escape from responsibility than it is a reality. But one could just as equally say that I chose to climb the tree and the fall with injury resulted from the law of gravity attendant on my carelessness or my poor decision. Since the choice was mine I am responsible for the outcome. As a cause-effect phenomenon the law of gravity provides impersonal feedback from which I can refine future choices - like not climbing trees. In this explanation there is no evasion of personal responsibility for the results of action taken.

> "You are the architect of your life and you decide your destiny."
> Swami Rama

84. Alter your way of evaluating what is real.

Keys to Contemplation

Spiritual Visioning
3. Alter your way of evaluating what is real.

- **Move away from beliefs, limited experience and outside authority!**
- **As projections, paradigms are self-fulfilling prophecies that continuously recreate your experience of reality.**
   Experimental feedback is the essence of a science.
- **Move to what you say is real, to what supports your highest vision from Spirit of what for you is personal mastery.**
   Dismiss all else as manifested illusion.

If the previous two shifts were difficult for the reader to cope with, this one will be even more difficult and has profound implications.

To suggest that the disciple move away from beliefs, experience and outside authority is a totally astonishing idea. The neuro-scientist, Karl Pribram, says that the brain structures experience in terms of what it is used to, in other words, in terms of past experience, what it has learned. We have said above that all your experience is structured by your model of the world - what you believe is real. That cognitive model acts like a mental filter that colours your experience of reality.

A simple analogy can be had with the pair of sunglasses. Put on green sunglasses and everything has a green tinge. If you did not know that you were wearing glasses (representing the belief systems that constitute models of the world which are subconscious and not part of ordinary awareness), you would think that you lived in a green reality. Yet this is simply a projection onto a neutral reality, through a filter which is the sunglasses.

A similar phenomenon can be demonstrated with hypnosis. Imagine for a minute that you are sitting in a room with several other people. You are in that room to get something so important that your life depends on it. The other people in the room are there to try to stop you from getting it. Now in your imagination look around the room at each of those other people and note the feelings you have about them and the meaning of the situation you find yourself in.

Now clap your hands together and stand up and walk for a minute to break that state.

Now sit down again and imagine that you are sitting in the same room with the same other people. Again you are in that room to get something so important that your life depends on it. But now everyone there will try to help you get what you want. Now in your imagination look around the room at each of those other people from this new position and note the difference in the feelings you have about them and about the meaning of the situation.

This simple exercise can help you understand how subconscious programming with beliefs can alter how you experience your world and how you will react to any given situation. Most aspects of models of the world are subconscious. You are not even aware of their action. Since you act from these experiences they create, then most of your manifesting comes by default.

Now the point is that beliefs are self-fulfilling prophecies because they are projections from a model of the world. They only let you see what you believe is there, what matches your belief system, and they can exclude the rest.

❈

Thus your experience continually verifies your beliefs over and over and you are locked into a self-fulfilling prophecy. To put it differently, you observe continually what is happening, and by giving your attention to it, focussing on it, you invite the universe to match that focus with more of the same. This cyclical phenomenon becomes habitual and can prevent the incremental change required on the spiritual path described in sutra 81. One simply makes the same mistakes over and over.

This phenomenon is often misunderstood by constructionists when they criticize positivistic science. What makes the scientific method so useful is not the hypothesis- or theory-making, but the hypothesis- or theory-testing. Reliable feedback from experiment - personal experience - is essential. If your beliefs do not match the data, (and you are sure the data are correct with no experimental error, using sound methodology, triangulation, etc.), then enlarge your beliefs and change your model of the world to include the new data. Regrettably most of us do not do this. We edit the data to sustain the belief system. Thus belief systems are homeostatic and very resistant to change.

In sutra 77 we discussed the paradigm shift and introduced the phrase, "My mind's made up, don't confuse me with facts." This is called the tomato effect in science (Jerry, 1985). The tomato effect refers to the confusion of theory with fact. It describes an inflexibility of mind in the face of new ideas that are at variance with current dogma.

> "The term was coined by Goodwin and Goodwin (1984) to describe an all too common situation in medicine where highly efficacious therapies can be ignored or rejected because they may not fit accepted theories of disease mechanism or drug action. A common version of the phenomenon is to think that because one has a logical or rational explanation for something it must be true. Despite the popularity of tomatoes in the continental European diet by the mid 16th century, this exotic fruit, which came originally from Peru, was shunned in North America. North Americans did not accept the tomato as even edible until the 1800's, and only during the past 80 years has the tomato become one of our largest commercial crops. According to the Goodwins (1984) the reason was obvious. Everyone knew that tomatoes were poisonous, since they belong to the nightshade (Solanaceae) family. The leaves and fruit of several members of the deadly nightshade family, such as belladonna or mandrake, can be fatal if taken in sufficient amounts. Only a fool would eat a tomato!"
> Jerry, 1985

If you cannot rely on your beliefs, experience or external authority, where is one to find truth? The answer is stunning! Move to what you say is real, as guided from your intuitions from the Centre of Consciousness, to what supports and contributes to your having mastery and to what supports and matches your highest vision from Spirit, from the Centre of Consciousness, of what for you is Heaven on Earth. Dismiss all else as manifested illusion.

Remember that you live out the past in the present in the sense that your current life situation is a manifestation of your previous model of the world. To manifest your new vision requires a strong, controlled, one-pointed mind that can hold the vision firmly despite the distractions coming from the current situation - a mind purified and honed by yogic practices of concentration and meditation.

Please note that this is not about stubbornness, forcing or personal willfulness. Nor is it about having to do it all alone by your own actions through struggle with a recalcitrant universe. Yes, you will perform plenty of action in the world as your vision manifests, but it will flow out of the inner prompting of the Centre of Consciousness in an ongoing dance with the synchronicities of a co-creative universal process.

85. *The universe restructures itself to fit your new models of reality.*

The universe, reality, mother nature, *prakriti*, *Shakti*, or Divine Mother (whatever term you may use) responds to your vibratory signal as you express intent for your vision through your new model of the world in your mind. It gives you more of what you habitually pay attention to. You experience that signal as a feeling, if not an actual emotion. Where you place your attention provides the signal to the universal co-creative process. The essence of your highest vision, which was given to you by Spirit, is embodied now in the values and beliefs that make up your new pictures of reality or model of the world in your mind. These values and beliefs, these contents of your model of the world, are very important to you. The universal co-creative process responds to your preoccupation, your fascination, where you place your attention, and its associated emotional signal - the positive feelings of inspiration that are associated with your vision. It then rearranges itself to accommodate this new model of reality. As you signal your intent by taking the first step toward your vision the universal cocreative process responds with a series of synchronicities that open almost magically to reveal the path moment by moment to the manifestation of your goal. The process unfolds with ease as you cooperate with it.

But note that you must take the first step to signal your strong intent and then the universe responds to you. Sitting around and waiting or wishing for something to happen in response to your wonderful ideas does not work. You are in charge; you have the choice; you initiate the co-creative process. Intentionality is everything, and you indicate you intent by making a decision, by acting, by taking the first step in faith with all of the risk that goes with it, by committing yourself.

To begin, use the mind to experiment with the three shifts above "as if" the vision were Truth, following your guidance from the Centre of Consciousness without hesitation. As the universal co-creative process begins to rearrange in response, you start to gain some supportive evidence and direct experience of the new ongoing manifestation. Since you approach this whole process as an experiment, you do not have to take the unfolding on blind faith. As a growing number of new supportive experiences that are consistent with the new manifestation arise then you experience a true yogic expanding faith. Like any science, the cocreative science is based in the evidence of the unfolding manifestation.

In the physical world of three dimensions there is inertia. Any change evolves gradually over time. Because of this inertia and gradual manifestation you will experience a transient "double exposure" of the new paradigm superimposed on the old as the latter fades and dies as a manifested illusion - atrophies from disuse since your attention which sustained it has now shifted to the new vision. The new reality will gradually come into being in validation of your vision.

86. Follow your Centre without wavering.

As your vision unfolds participate wholeheartedly and do your part as you feel guided by Spirit from the Centre of Consciousness. Follow that guidance without hesitation. As the universal co-creative process rearranges itself to accommodate your new vision of reality you will automatically participate in, be involved with, and be transformed by this process.

Your new vision sets the transpersonal background reality, your true identity as someone who has mastery of the co-creative process. You are now a transpersonal entity identified with and expressing the Centre of Consciousness, on a transpersonal mission in service of humankind in the spirit of true Karma Yoga. The various roles that you will play in the foreground will take care of themselves. You will live as an element in the foreground with the fullness and magnificence of who you are in day-to-day life as a personal instrument for divine expression.

Your vision is always of the end result, the what, and not the how. You leave the process, the how, up to Spirit and abandon any fear and your need to control. As you manifest your vision have no attachment to anything in the world of form - to people, to places, to things, to emotions, to ideas or to concepts - to how things should or ought to be. The background reality will determine what the foreground reality is like. The only source of struggle and conflict in a life lived this way is having desires which conflict with Spirit, with your Centre of Consciousness. Align your desires and the parts of your personality completely with Spirit; act with integrity (sutra 49) This kind of alignment is meant when words like "surrender", "harmony", or "yogic purification" are used. It means to be so aligned vibrationally with your vision that it feels so real, so inevitable, as though it already exists as a certainty. It is not a matter of whether it will manifest, but simply when. And you have full faith that the "when" will come in right timing. This is what is referred to as pure intent flowing from the Centre of Consciousness. This way you and Spirit each put the same things into the manifestation process so that your life is powerful and without struggle.

87. Karma Yoga is action flowing from the Centre of Consciousness.

When your vision manifests, then create a higher one. Move through progressive iterations of visioning until your version of the highest that you can be becomes fully manifested. Rather than being a selfish exercise of the ego this process of visioning is a channelling of Spirit's vision for the co-creation of "Heaven on Earth", a divine manifestation for which you become the instrument in surrender to your divine core or Centre of Consciousness. Your unfolding as a master comes through being a skilled and aligned instrument for this process of divine manifestation, in perfect surrender to your divine core.

> "Our Father, who art in heaven,
> Hallowed be thy name.
> Thy kingdom come.
> Thy will be done on earth as it is in heaven. ..."
> The Lord's Prayer

This becomes the essence of Karma Yoga. Before the Centre of Consciousness opens as a direct inner experience one follows the rules laid down for Karma Yoga, including selfless service and surrender of the fruits of action to the divine. But once the Centre of Consciousness becomes a living inner experience and action begins to flow naturally from that Centre, true Karma Yoga becomes one's natural expression rather than just following some rules.

Action that is based on intent from the Centre of Consciousness does not create personal karma in the same way as action that flows from the ego. You find yourself flowing naturally and easily with events, always doing the right thing with the right people in the right place at the right time and in the right way. This concept of right action is an integral part of divine expression. Yoga is truly skill in action.

We have mentioned purity of intent. We might also use the words "will" or "desire" for intent. One way to think of purity of intent is to realize that a mind trained in meditation is a powerful creative instrument. It is based in one-pointedness. When this kind of uninterrupted, one-pointed focus is used to visualize, the creative process becomes very powerful. There are no interrupting thoughts or background noise to dilute the purity of the intent and focus. In particular, there are no objectors or resistances to weaken the co-creative process. Each time a thought of "yes but ...." arises in the mind, it dilutes, weakens and confuses the purity of the vibrational signal which is sent out by the intent. Like any vibrational energy phenomenon these positive and negative signals add algebraically. If one transmits a creative signal that is confused, having desires mixed with resistances, the universal co-creative process can only respond with a confused manifestation, if indeed the mixed signal is not totally neutralized so that nothing can manifest. Thus purity of intent and powerful creation mean a fully aligned and coherent expression of will using a one-pointed focus by a mind trained in the disciplines of concentration and meditation. A modern and particularly lucid presentation of the ideas discussed here may be found in Hicks and Hicks (1998; 1991), but the concepts are as old as the yoga science.

Another way to think of purity of intent is in terms of commitment and alignment. Co-creation is most powerful when all parts of the personality are aligned with the intent from the Centre of Consciousness so that there are no psychological objectors or resistance. The result is total commitment to the action. For an advanced disciple who has meditation skills and some mental control any feelings of hesitancy about an action to be performed should raise a red flag of warning. If these resistances cannot be resolved then one should consider not moving forward with the action planned, so that something negative that is not wanted does not materialize.

> "Until one is committed there is hesitancy, the chance to draw back, always ineffectiveness. Concerning all acts of initiative (and creation), there is one elementary truth, the ignorance of which kills countless ideas and splendid plans: that the moment one definitely commits oneself (makes a decision), then Providence moves too. All sorts of things happen to help one that

would not otherwise have occurred. A whole stream of events issues from the decision, raising in one's favour all manner of unforeseen incidents and meetings and material assistance, which no man could have dreamt would come his way ... Whatever you can do, or dream you can, begin it. Boldness has genius, power and magic in it."
Johann Wolfgang von Goethe

What Goethe has described here, of course, is synchronicity. The adept learns to recognize and to work with serendipity and synchronicity. In the West we take these two to be the products of chance, good fortune. Indeed they are not. Their appearance represents the universal co-creative process in action. Both favour the prepared mind. The mind is prepared by careful attention to the visioning process and its construction. The interaction of the two results in recognition of the unfolding universal process. The individual has an internal sense of the right action, the right steps to take at any moment in the process as each synchronicity presents itself, and the doors open smoothly toward the manifestation of the vision. Struggle, forcing things, and exhausting personal action and doing are the antithesis of this process. If you are struggling to make something work then you are not using the co-creative process properly. Most likely the intent is not pure and there is not full commitment and alignment with what is wanted. The Inner Teacher, the Centre of Consciousness, plays a key role in this process.

Sri Aurobindo had this to say:

> "All developed mental men, those who get beyond the average, have in one way or other, or it least at certain times and for certain purposes, to separate the two parts of the mind, the active part, which is a factory of thoughts and the quiet masterful part which is at once a Witness and a Will, observing them, judging, rejecting, eliminating, accepting, ordering corrections and changes, the Master in the House of Mind."
Aurobindo 1972, p83.

The Mother, Sri Aurobindo's partner, was a great yogini in her own right. With regard to the actions of synchronicity she had the following comments:

> "If you have within you ... (an inner Being) ... sufficiently awake to watch over you, to prepare your path, it can draw towards you things which help you, draw people, books, circumstances, all sorts of little coincidences which come to you as though brought by some benevolent will and give you an indication, a help, a support to take decisions and turn you in the right direction. But once you have taken this decision, once you have decided to find the truth of your being, once you start sincerely on the road, then

everything seems to conspire to help you in your advance."
The Mother, 1972, p233

These quotations refer to how the universe reorganizes itself to fit your models of reality, and the role played by the Centre in this process. One should realize that the guidance can be both external as well as internal. We have described the internal guidance in the form of the intuitive whisperings directly from the Centre, initially when the mind is still in meditation, and later at any time the devotee wishes to remember. External guidance comes as described in the quotations above with the many synchronicities and serendipities that appear. Sometimes help comes from the most unlikely sources and unlikely people. We have even had books we needed to read fall off a shelf at our feet in a section of a bookstore where they would never have been found had we been looking for them deliberately, because they had been misfiled. Individuals and circumstances become instruments, so to speak, to deliver parts of the universal response to your creating.

And what of commitment? It has been said that in a North American breakfast of bacon and eggs, the chicken is involved, but the pig is committed!

Meditation

88. With the opening of the Centre of Consciousness meditation moves from method to experience, from doing to being, from effort to absorption.

The popular presentation of yoga, and especially meditation, emphasizes its healing and anti-stress effects. In the beginning this is so, particularly when it is used only for its therapeutic effects. But when spiritual *sadhana* is undertaken seriously, the going soon gets rough as the process of purification begins in earnest. There is a general consensus among transpersonal psychologists that one needs a healthy ego to undertake serious spiritual *sadhana* (Washburn, 1995; Wilber, 1996). Psychological stresses occur during the beginning and intermediate stages of the practice. Yoga often attracts individuals who are looking for a solution for personal problems or as a substitute for psychological therapy. The student who brings immaturity, poor ego development or poor adjustment in general to the practice may actually find his or her problems becoming worse.

When the mind begins to internalize during meditation (or what is really concentration in the beginning), the lid comes off the unconscious mind and its repressed material begins to surface (Walsh, 1979). Repressed feelings like anger, hostility, fear, sadness, grief, depression, etc. must be faced without your being overwhelmed by them. The upsurge of unconscious material and threats to physical balance can be intensified with the extensive use of a purificatory mantra like Gayatri in the context of a *purashcharana*, which, therefore, should only be undertaken under the close supervision of an experienced teacher of meditation. Despite years of intensive spiritual work Ram Dass, for example, had to face episodes of serious emotional disturbance for which he found psychotherapy was helpful (Alpert/Ram Dass, 1982). The serious student should have access to competent medical and psychological help as required during intense *sadhana*. Such professional help should be knowledgeable about and sympathetic to spiritual *sadhana* (Nelson, 1994). The aspirant should become familiar with the dissociative processes associated with the witnessing state that produce the visual-kinesthetic dissociation that is a principal way by which meditation purifies the mind. The new "power therapies" or meridian energy psychologies may prove to be potent aids for easing the emotional turbulence that can sometimes accompany sadhana (Gallo, 1999).

With the opening of the Centre of Consciousness comes both challenge and relief. On the one hand the *sadhana* now intensifies under the guidance of the Inner Teacher. The discipline becomes more exacting. It can be a greater challenge physically and mentally to maintain detachment and balance. Attention to diet, exercise and stress management become very important: the regulation of the four urges of sleep, sex, food and self-preservation (ie stress). The process becomes demanding and all-consuming like the training of an elite athlete or concert artist. But on the other hand, the Centre increasingly becomes an anchor of peace, stillness and security around which the storm of purification rages. The awareness can be anchored into the Centre by constant remembrance to provide a stable point of reference and strength for the achievement of balance in the midst of the storm. The ability to endure becomes important and this stems from the acquisition of great faith and patience through being firmly anchored in the Centre.

Meditation is still the principal access to the awareness of the Centre. But more and more it moves from being a process or a set of methods and techniques rooted in a need for action, doing and accomplishment, to one of surrender to being and direct experience. To be in the storm is to struggle and maintain balance in a place where forces push one into reactivity to the turbulence of the purification. To move into the still point is more like moving from the storm itself into the metaphoric eye of the hurricane where the stillness and detachment can bring some succour to the harried soul as the storm whirls about without.

89. With the opening of the Centre of Consciousness meditation moves from activity to communion, to at-one-ment.

Keys to Contemplation

- Meditation is both method and state of consciousness.
- To shift your identity means to move from doing to being.
- By communion is meant loving relationship; but At-one-ment goes beyond to Oneness.

We think of meditation as a method, as a set of instructions to follow for an internal mental practice, perhaps because this is how we are initially taught it. We learn to experience meditation as doing. Yet we are also told that meditation is a state of awareness, a state of consciousness, a state of being. When we are taught to meditate, we are really being taught to concentrate. We are told that the state of meditation will flow from perfect concentration spontaneously, and, well, *samadhi* is somewhere far beyond.

> "Dharana means confinement of the mind to one point or one object or one area. ... if you are concentrating on a mantra there should be awareness of it throughout, without a break. If there is a break it is concentration; if there is no break it becomes meditation or dhyana. ... In concentration there is always awareness that you are concentrating. Meditation is not different from concentration. It is a higher quality of it. ... In dharana there is awareness of the object, which is broken from time to time in the process. Dhyana includes two things: one, an unbroken continuous flow of consciousness of the single object, and two, the awareness that you are practising unbroken concentration. If in dharana the consciousness becomes continuous so that there is no break or interruption due to any other thought, then dharana is replaced by or turned into dhyana. ... In dhyana there is an uninterrupted flow of consciousness. However, in samadhi, you do not remain aware of your own existence, there is not even the awareness that you are practising concentration. Thus there are two characteristics of samadhi: one, the object alone shines and two, there is no awareness of the process or of the self. ... [The process] starts with a subjective and objective awareness; that is a dual awareness. You are aware of your object of meditation within as well as in the outside world, but gradually the outer doors are closed and you see only the thing that is inside. That is dhyana. Then the thing seen inside becomes clearer and clearer and simultaneously you lose your personal consciousness, that is called samadhi. The three put together are known as samyama."
> Swami Satyananda Saraswati, 1989, pp 231-236.

As beginning meditators in the West we have to have an answer to the question "how?" Paradoxically we are instructed in a method, in doing, as a means to gain a state of being. One cannot just tell someone to be in a particular way if that internal state is unknown to them. Most of us cannot go to certain inner states at will, and certainly not to inner states that are unknown, that have never been experienced. So how is this to be achieved? One gives the student a method, a set of instructions for action. One can tell people what to do but one cannot tell them how to be. Communicating the how is the biggest challenge. Be peaceful! But how? Be loving! But how? Being and doing are antitheses, and yet each can generate the other. The synthesis of this duality lies at the basis of the practice - to use it as doing (mixed with a generous portion of grace) to find the experience of the still point within, and then to reverse the process by acting from this still point. Whether as a practice or as a state, meditation is the essence of it all. But when the Centre of Consciousness dominates one can go to It at will and find those states within It. The process becomes something we all can do, which is simply to remember that Presence. Constant remembering of the Presence that is the Centre becomes meditation in action.

In sutra 82 we talked about shifting your identity. This identity shift is a move from doing to being. The ego certainly experiences internal states ranging from self awareness through kinesthetics to emotions. Because it is grounded in the manifest personality the states are always shifting in the ego's experience. Thus there is always the experience of action and doing: shifting activity at the physical level, shifting thoughts at the mental level, and shifting feelings at the emotional level. And all of this occurs in a changing external environmental context. Change, movement and time are fundamental to the experience of living in manifested reality. However, the identity shift to the Centre of Consciousness lifts the core identification of self from the ego as doer to the Centre of Consciousness as foundational Being; from the changing to the changeless; from finite time with its past and future to the infinite internal Now; from the agitation of activity to the peace of being - the *shanti*, the peace that passes all understanding; from confusion (*avidya*) to clarity (*vidya*). The sun finally breaks through the clouds of the mental landscape.

By communion is meant loving relationship - I and Thou, I and THAT. By At-one-ment is meant going beyond the duality of relationship to oneness - I am THAT, and eventually, All is THAT: there is only THAT. From THAT arises all and into THAT all subsides again. One acts in the world of manifestation, but one exists in Being. Manifestation is a derivative state; Being is the fundamental State.

90. The three-fold distinctions of subject-object consciousness collapse into the unity of absorption.

Keys to Contemplation

- **In samsara knowing comes through subject-object consciousness.**
- **In the Now of the Centre of Consciousness Knowing reduces to Consciousness-Without-An-Object.**
- **The transition from dharana and dhyana to samadhi is from knowing about to pure Knowing Itself.**
- **The identity shift is from ego to Centre, from cognition about to pure Awareness Itself, which is absorption.**

To live in the manifested world is to live in duality. Cognition occurs in subject-object consciousness. Knowing is always knowing-about, consciousness-with-an-object. The object is experienced as a mental object, content or sensory stimulation. To know (cognition) is to know something. There is a three fold distinction of knower (*grahitr*), the object of experience to be known (*grahya*) and the instrument of knowing (*grahana*), which includes the fact and the process, as well as the means of experiencing and cognizing (Arya, 1986, p188). These distinctions are not just philosophical constructs. With the opening of the Centre the aspirant will learn to observe the mind with detachment and to make these distinctions in particular cases. This process of discernment also produces *vairagya*, detachment towards the particular object or experience in point.

In contrast, however, the Now of the inner Presence that is the Centre of Consciousness presents a very different experience where knowing reduces to Consciousness-Without-An-Object. Here we are using Merrell-Wolff's terminology (1994). Awareness focussed in the Centre is transcendent. In contrast to the experience of duality, of knowledge about, one can never exhaust the potential of the knowing, especially in language. The three-fold distinctions of subject-object consciousness collapse into a pure Knowing Itself. There is a move from incomplete and potentially erroneous knowing about something to direct intuitive apperception of that knowing itself, as though that knowing and the object or experience to which it refers were oneself. There is no longer the experience of a knowing, a process of knowing and an object or experience to be known, but only pure knowing itself, leading eventually to pure awareness, pure Consciousness, Consciousness-Without-An-Object.

> "... The direct value of that Recognition (Consciousness-without-an-object) is inexpressible and inconceivable in the sense of concepts meaning just what they are defined to mean and no more. Of necessity, all concepts deal with content in some sense, as they are born in the tension of a subject aware of objects and refer to objects. Consciousness-without-an-object is not an object on the level where it is realized. But just as soon as words are employed to refer to it, we have in place of the actual reality a sort of shadowy reflection. This reflection may be useful as a symbol pointing toward the Reality, but becomes a deception just as soon as it is regarded as a comprehensive concept. Conceivable conclusions may be derived from the original symbol, but the full realization of That which is symbolized requires the dissolving of the very power of representation itself."
>
> Merrell-Wolff, 1994, p315.

The transition from concentration and meditation to absorption, from *dharana/dhyana* to *samadhi*, is a movement from hearing about things or ideas or objects to a state of pure knowing itself. It should now be clear from the discussion of this sutra that the transition from meditation to *sabija samadhi* (absorption) involves collapse of subject-object consciousness; both the knower and the process of knowing disappear and only the object of knowing shines forth. The transition to *nirbija samadhi* is then to Consciousness-Without-An-Object.

Clearly the identity shift discussed in sutra 82 is also the same transition, ultimately from subject-object consciousness to Consciousness-Without-An-Object. The identity shift moves from the ego to the Centre of Consciousness. It moves from cognition about something to pure awareness itself, which is absorption. In the initial awareness of the Centre in meditation the meditator will sense the mantra in the background while the intensity of the Centre becomes foreground and seems to reach out with its bliss to absorb the awareness. This experience can be frightening and when that fear suddenly arises the meditator will lose the Centre. If one can surrender and allow the awareness to dissolve into that Centre, then the Centre is not lost but becomes intensified or expanded.

Thus meditation is both process and a state. Meditation is key to working with the Centre of Consciousness and for the identity shift to occur.

91. *Meditation gradually becomes spontaneous.*

Keys to Contemplation

- **The identity shifts from self to Self.**
- **Meditation shifts from process to internal state.**

Another way to say this is that one's focus of consciousness, one's internal locus of control, one's centre or point of personal reference, one's sense of core identity, shifts more and more into identification with the Centre of Consciousness as its basis and foundation rather than with the shifting and changing ego. Because the Centre of Consciousness is changeless, this brings stability and increasing peacefulness to the personality no matter how it may be beset by personal or external circumstances.

This is also another way to describe the identity shift discussed above. It is also another way to describe the shift in meditation from process to internal state.

Note that this is not a description of enlightenment. We are dealing here only with the entry to the true Path. It is only the beginning of the higher life.

> "Meditation will give you the capacity to improve your health, your relationships and the skillfulness of all your activities. This is because meditation can do something that no other technique can accomplish - it introduces you to yourself on all levels, and finally leads you to the Centre of Consciousness within."
> Swami Rama, 1992

92. *There are yogas of life and yogas of discipline.*

Swami Veda Bharati classifies yogas as the yogas of life and the yogas of discipline (figure 4, p169). The yogas of life are three: Bhakti Yoga is the yoga of devotion; Jnana Yoga is the yoga of wisdom; and the yoga of action is Karma Yoga. They are called yogas of life since they operate in everyday living as a lifestyle. The aspirant tends to specialize in one according to the dominant features of his or her personality (Swami Rama, 1982b). Each of these paths has a central text. These texts are not necessarily exclusive; the Gita, for example, discusses all of these paths.

The yogas of life, however, are grounded in Raja Yoga (The Royal

168 Sutras of the Inner Teacher

Path) as the foundation. Within Raja Yoga there are component paths of specialization, one or more of which may be assigned at different stages of *sadhana* by the teacher. These might be considered as chapters in the book of Raja Yoga. Thus Raja Yoga makes up the yogas of discipline. The core text for Raja Yoga is the *Yogasutras* of Patanjali, where the component eight limbs are described in *padas* II and III (Aranya, 1981). Since eight steps or limbs make up Raja yoga, it is also called *Ashtanga* (eight-limbed) yoga. The first five steps are the external limbs, while the last three are the internal limbs. Hatha yoga proper comprises the first four steps. All paths up the mountain lead to the same view at the top. There is a link between the yogas of life and the eight-fold path. Step seven is meditation which is the foundational technique for all paths. Even those practising the yogas of life still do some form of meditation.

All of the yogas become integrated into the realization of the Centre of Consciousness. One ends up effectively practising all three of the yogas of life to some degree on a foundation of Raja Yoga, even though one may specialize in a particular yoga of life and/or subdiscipline within Raja Yoga. People are individuals; the wise teacher finds plenty of room to tailor an evolving prescription for *sadhana* to meet the needs of the individual student.

All three of the yogas of life have been discussed above in the context of the Centre of Consciousness. The process of unceasing worship with devotion is Bhakti Yoga (sutras 65 and 69 - 75). The unfolding of intuition with its interactive communication with the Centre of Consciousness is a phase of Jnana Yoga (sutras 54 and 55). The expression of the Centre of Consciousness into action is Karma Yoga (sutras 76 through 87). Although the *Ashtanga* yoga of Patanjali is shown as a serial process, in fact the steps become simultaneous. The importance of the *yamas* and *niyamas* as moral precepts has been emphasized above under the concept of qualification (*adhikara*). All of the yogas culminate in *samadhi*. Although the *Yogasutras* do not directly refer to the *kundalini*, we show the point of its awakening in figure 4, which leads to expansion of consciousness in meditation into *samadhi*. The energy of successful concentration that explodes the *bindu* ignites the serpent force.

Although this is perhaps a simplistic classification of the yogas, we believe it to be a practical and useful map for the aspirant. We have not discussed Vedanta or Tantra here, which lead to even more encompassing maps.

93. Meditation is the beginning and the end of all of these.

"... meditation can do something that no other technique can accomplish - it introduces you to yourself on all levels, and finally leads you to the Centre of

SAMADHI
(Self-Realization, turiya, 4th state)

◄ Siddhis (powers)
◄ Awakening of Kundalini

INTERNAL LIMBS

DHYANA
(Meditation)

DHARANA
(Concentration)

PRATYAHARA
(Control of Senses)

PRANAYAMA
(Breath Control)

ASANA
(Posture)

NIYAMA
(Observances)

YAMA
(Restrictions)

HATHA YOGA

EXTERNAL LIMBS

YOGAS OF LIFE

BHAKTI YOGA (Devotion)
(Bhakti Sutras)

JNANA YOGA (Wisdom)
(Upanishads, Brahma Sutras)

KARMA YOGA
Bhagavad Gita)

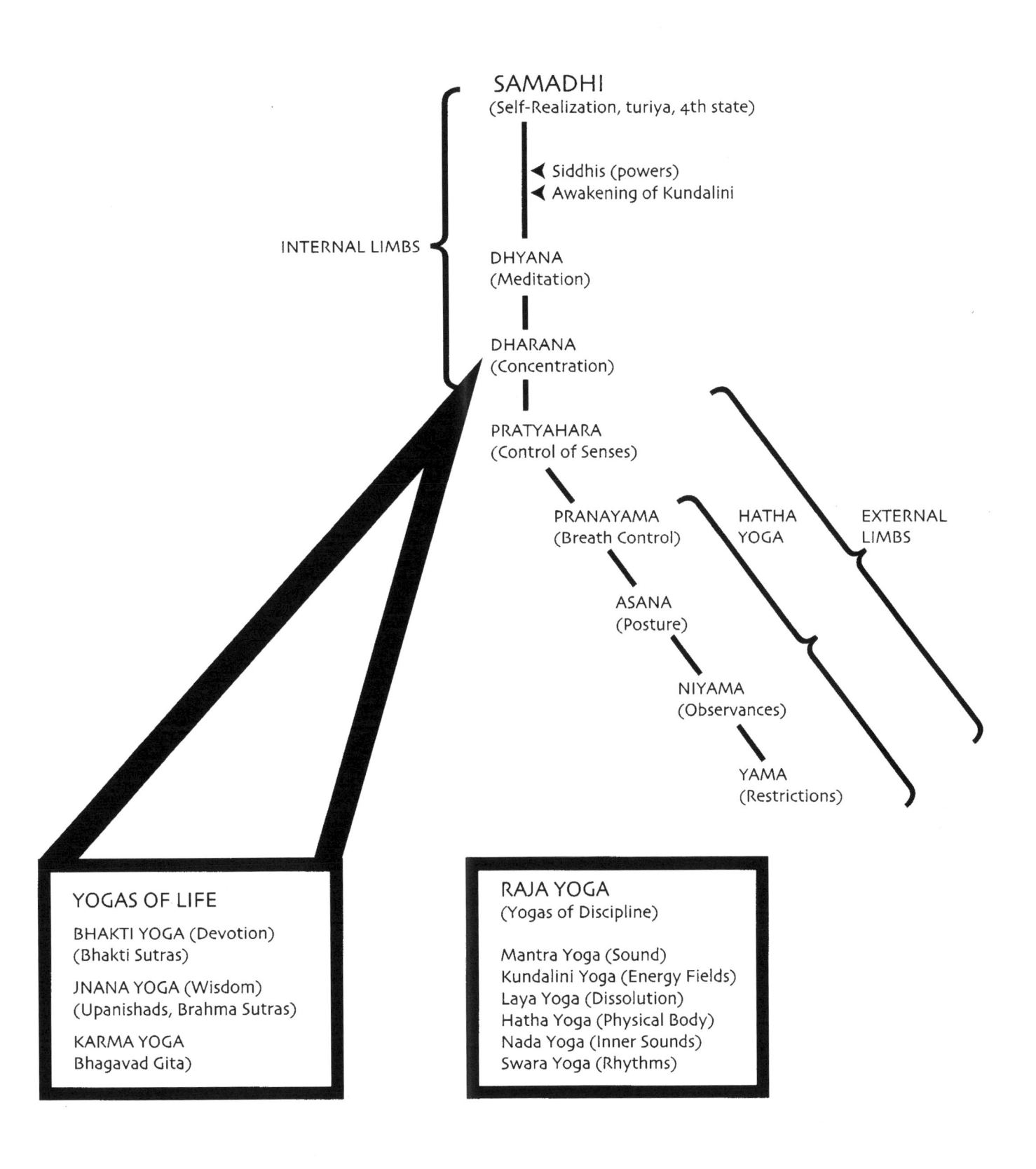

RAJA YOGA
(Yogas of Discipline)

Mantra Yoga (Sound)
Kundalini Yoga (Energy Fields)
Laya Yoga (Dissolution)
Hatha Yoga (Physical Body)
Nada Yoga (Inner Sounds)
Swara Yoga (Rhythms)

Figure 4. The Yogas of Life and Discipline

> Consciousness within, from where consciousness flows on various degrees and levels. This Centre of Consciousness is called Atman. The seeker's aspirations are fulfilled when he or she becomes fully aware of Atman, the inner dweller, and then no longer identifies with the objects of the mind and the world."
>
> Swami Rama, 1992, p xi

Meditation is the core technique for yoga as the science of spirituality, and for the spiritual path. In sutra 65 we discussed the chariot of *sadhana*, with its two simultaneous wheels of *abhyasa* and *vairagya*. Meditation is the essential method for *abhyasa*, attunement and at-one-ment with the Centre of Consciousness. At the same time, meditation is also the core technique for purifying the mind to produce detachment (*vairagya*), in part through its production of visual-kinesthetic dissociation.

As we approach the New Age at the time of the second millennium, much is being written about "ascension". Whether one interprets this to mean enlightenment in the traditional sense of yoga or to refer to raising personal and planetary vibration in the context of a major planetary transition, the practices are much the same and some form of meditation remains central. Meditation underlies the ability to attune with the Centre in love and worship (Bhakti Yoga) and for intuitive inner teaching and guidance (Jnana Yoga). It also underlies the ability to discern the Centre's intent to express in continuous co-creative action (Karma Yoga) in daily living. Meditation places one in the centre of one's life contract or mission so that one is always engaged in right action. In short, it spiritualizes and optimizes daily life. Thus meditation is the engine of purification which drives the chariot of *sadhana* with its two wheels of *abhyasa* and *vairagya*, in which the identity rides to shift into Self-Realization with its co-creative expression into action as service in the world.

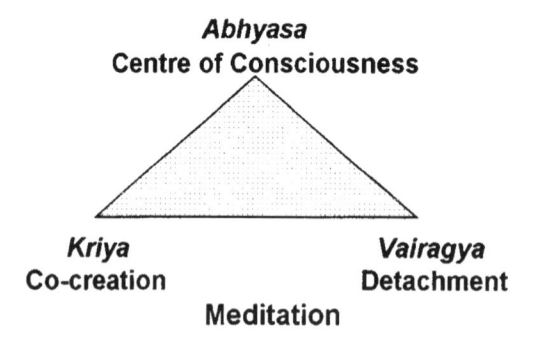

Abhyasa
Centre of Consciousness

Kriya   **Vairagya**
Co-creation   **Detachment**
Meditation

The Tradition of the Himalayan Masters is an initiatory tradition. Initiation, beginning with a personal mantra, is an essential step for the aspirant on this path to begin to establish the link of his or her consciousness with the

Inner Teacher, a link that comes to full fruition later with higher initiations if the seed of the personal mantra is nourished with faithful practice. Seeds planted in a garden come to fruition when the gardener keeps the garden weeded and provides for fertilization, air, water and sunshine. Meditation is the foundational technique for working with that spiritual seed that has been implanted through initiation. The Himalayan Tradition is an ancient lineage. It is said that this Tradition contains within it and can be traced back as the origin, of all authentic paths of meditation; all other paths have merged from it. It is the trunk and roots of the tree of *sadhana* and all other paths are its branches.

94. *There are as many Paths as there are Pilgrims.*

We have described four main paths of yoga: the three yogas of life and the eight-fold path of *Ashtanga* yoga with its subvariants in sutra 92. People agonize over which path to choose. Swami Rama has addressed this important choice in detail (Swami Rama, 1982b). Some agonize so much they move from path to path, expression to expression, collecting techniques, experiences, initiations and mantras as they go, but they never progress. Like someone who wants to be a medical doctor, such individuals do the equivalent of taking first year medicine in school after school, comparing each as they go to try to logically find the best curriculum. But they never graduate! Initially a student may sample many traditions and many expressions of a particular tradition, drinking a little of the cup of each. But eventually the serious student must settle into one tradition and dig that well deep in order to succeed.

Digging the well deep does not mean being doctrinaire and exclusive. It means having a home base, absorbing that particular world view of the teachings deeply, and using those methods to develop expertise and form that set of grooves in the personality that build energetic pathways to superconsciousness with reliability and control. It does not mean becoming close-minded to any expression of yoga other than one's own tradition, teachings and doctrine. Swami Rama's master sent him to study with many sages. At the annual Congress of the Himalayan Institute in Honesdale he invited many speakers to represent different views and traditions; all had an honoured place in the program to express their view of Truth. Students were encouraged to study widely and to question critically. The objective was not indoctrination, but to develop in the student the ability to discriminate the Truth of the one Spirit in whatever guise It presents. This discrimination tends to become diluted in generations removed from the master with the development of rigid doctrine and ritual used with the dress and trappings of yoga.

Yet in the face of all of this we say there are as many paths as those who choose to walk a path. How can that be? Consider the following metaphor.

In sutra 92 we presented the major paths up to the top of the mountain of spirituality. By whatever route one climbs, the view is the same from the top - all paths eventually lead to the summit. Some paths up the mountain are long and gradual; others are rapid and precipitous - all according to the intent and qualification of the aspirant.

Yet in taking any of these main paths, each journey is still unique. How is this so?

Some go alone and some go with friends; some go in the morning, some in the afternoon, some in the evening, and some with the moonlight and stars at night; some travel with the new life of spring, others in the heat of the summer, some with the colours of fall, and some through the white of winter; some travel in the rain while others travel in the heat of the sun; some are bundled against the cold while others sweat with the heat; some meet wildlife on the way, some are bothered by insects, some experience none of these; some travel with enthusiasm and others not; some walk with experience but some are novices to hiking; some are well-equipped while others walk unencumbered; some begin their journey impulsively while others carefully plan ahead. One could go on and on.

Yet each reaches the same sign posts: a particular promontory with a special view; a particular patch of woods; a particular large rock by the path; a particular bridge to be crossed over a bubbling stream; perhaps a direction sign or some paint marks on the rocks or blazes cut on the trees to point the way.

And yet all end up at the same place at the top of the mountain. Having walked the same physical path up the mountain each has had a unique experience.

The particular version of the spiritual path taught by a particular master will reflect his or her experience. A particular version will be more or less helpful to various types of students and hence influence their choice of a particular method. There are many masters, and vive la difference! Beware therefore of thinking that your path and master hold the only version of truth, however right and appropriate it may be for you. Allow others to choose their way and be ready to offer your experience as stimulation to their own intuitions, but not as a misguided attempt to proselytize. For ultimately the choice of the path and the journey itself are a unique co-creation of the student with Spirit under the guidance of the Inner Teacher. Honour that unique co-creation. A true teacher facilitates this self-discovery and empowerment for each of his or her students, rather than prescribing a rigid doctrine and ritual as the only way. Yoga is a spiritual science, and true science is neither dogmatic nor doctrinaire. The wisdom of its discovery grows through the feedback of experience as it progresses towards truth.

95. *The mantram comes from and goes back to the Centre of Consciousness*

Keys to Contemplation

- **Mantra initiation comes from the Centre of Consciousness.**
- **The mantra leads the aspirant back to the Centre of Consciousness.**
- **Initiation formally connects the aspirant to the yoga tradition.**

Initiators are empowered by the guru or master to give mantra initiation as the first initiatory step in the tradition. The initiator and student meditate together, and in deep meditation the initiator "hears" the personal or guru mantra appropriate for the student and then whispers it into the student's right ear, giving instructions on how to use it. Although the actual mantras may be found in the texts (e.g. Swami Satyananda Saraswati, 1975; Swami Vishnu Devananda, 1978), this is a revelatory process from the Centre of Consciousness. An energetic seed is implanted into the aspirant's mental field. If the aspirant nurtures that seed by steady, correct practice of mantra meditation, it gradually flourishes, becoming the grace and gift of the Inner Teacher that will eventually guide the aspirant home, back to its source in the Centre of Consciousness. The personal mantra comes from, is revealed by, the Centre and eventually returns to the Centre.

The mantra is like the light from a lighthouse, penetrating the darkness of ignorance and guiding the spiritual Pilgrim back to the safety of port.

The Himalayan Tradition is an initiatory tradition. To use an approximate analogy, the aspirant is like a metal needle placed in contact with a powerful magnet - the spiritual master. When the needle is separated it is permanently changed by magnetization, and now carries some of that magnetic property as its own, and as its attraction to the magnetism of the source. The link to the Tradition whose source is the Centre of Consciousness, is through mantra initiation. It is the step that formally starts the aspirant on this path.

96. In the Centre of Consciousness love, wisdom and action are unified.

Keys to Contemplation

- **Love, wisdom and action are unified in the Centre of Consciousness.**
- **One's sadhana reflects all three.**

You have all seen a diamond glittering in the sunlight. Each of its facets reflects the light differently. As you view it from different angles it seems to flash different colours of the light spectrum in turn. First red, then tones of orange and yellow; then green moving into hues of blue, indigo and violet - each hue an aspect of the unity of white light itself.

So it is with the Centre of Consciousness, except that the Centre is self-effulgent and does not reflect some secondary source. The "light" of the metaphor above becomes the different varieties and grades of Consciousness. At one moment it projects love and bliss, at another the flash of intuition; yet again it flows with intent to action. All of these - love, wisdom and will - become unified in the Centre of Consciousness. All of the yogas of life are unified in the Centre of Consciousness. At this stage the aspirant practices a mix of all three, a mix that varies from time to time, unified in the loving dance between disciple and master, between individual consciousness and the Inner Teacher.

97. From the Centre of Consciousness flow both witnessing awareness and awareness with intent.

Keys to Contemplation

- **Cultivate the Internal Witness.**
- **The Internal Witness is an expression of the Centre of Consciousness.**
- **The Witness is the foundation of mental equanimity.**
- **The Witness is the foundation of a one-pointed mind.**

There is much talk about the *sakshi*, the internal Witness, in discussions of meditation and yoga. With the opening of the Centre of Consciousness the internal Witness becomes an experienced reality.

On a one hand, the experience is a static, still, unmoving witnessing or watching of the mind, the emotions, and actions - a background Presence. It is a key state to achieving the mental purification and detachment by the process of visual-kinesthetic dissociation that underlies meditation and such meditative processes as *antar mouna* (Swami Satyananda Saraswati, 1975). Stabilization of that awareness, which is a partial expression of the Centre of Consciousness, becomes meditation in action. It is a very high state of Consciousness that lends stability and equanimity to the mind (Kristof and Emami, 1999). It is like the energy of a spinning top that spins so fast it appears to be still and motionless, yet it is perfectly balanced.

Aequanimitas

"Thou must be like a promontory of the sea, against which, though the waves beat continually, yet it both itself stands, And about it are those swelling waves stilled and quieted."
Marcus Aurelius

"In the physician or surgeon no quality takes rank with Imperturbability."
Sir William Osler

"The trouble with Archie is he don't know how to worry without gettin' upset!"
Television Character, Edith Bunker

Detachment and nonattachment are more rich concepts than mere objectivity and yet they include these. But this Presence is a state of consciousness that has the properties of detachment or nonattachment, and is not just simply these alone. It is an expression of the Centre of Consciousness as a new quality of inner space.

Yet paradoxically from this still, witnessing state also flows the subtlest, purest intent and will to action. It guides the mental focus in co-creation. It is the foundation of the one-pointed mind, for the essence of the one-pointed mind is absolute stillness and silence as the context for that point of focus in the Presence.

98. *Surrender all practice to the Centre of Consciousness.*

Keys to Contemplation

- **Perform all action surrendered to the Centre of Consciousness.**
- **Only *sadhana* done with awareness of the Centre of Consciousness is truly fruitful.**
- **Surrender stabilized is meditation in action.**
- **The flow of wisdom from the Internal Teacher becomes continuous.**
- **The identity shift completes itself into stable transpersonal awareness.**

With the opening of the Centre of Consciousness, all *sadhana* is done immersed in the awareness of that Centre and flows into action effortlessly from It. Indeed, the practice becomes to live all life within Its awareness and flowing from It. This is to surrender all practice to the Centre of Consciousness.

Yoga postures flow from It; breathing is done from It; meditation moves into It; daily thought, speech and actions flow from It. Only *sadhana* done with Its awareness bears real fruit; *sadhana* done mechanically from habit without this awareness is effort largely wasted and is perhaps only ten percent beneficial (The Mother, 1979). As this surrender becomes complete, as the awareness stabilizes, then there is constant meditation in action. This is the ultimate in pedagogy. To be aware of the Centre of Consciousness in all things is to listen silently for its wordless guidance, wisdom and intuition; a state of moment by moment flow of teaching that illumines life and action in all things.

Eventually that awareness becomes so stable and pervasive that the distinction between the small self as ego and that larger awareness blurs. The identity shifts and one's normal awareness becomes transpersonal.

99. *Life becomes a living meditation.*

Sri Aurobindo is best known among the sages of modern India for bringing yoga into active life in the world. Like the Himalayan Tradition, his Integral or purna yoga is not done to release the soul from matter into a higher transcendence, but to bring spirit into biology, to integrate and spiritualize the mind-body system at all levels. His supramental yoga then completes the transformation by bringing down into human experience the full energy and supreme knowledge (gnosis) of the Divine. (To Aurobindo, God was the Mother, the feminine expression of the Divine. In Sri Vidya, a very advanced tantric practice in the Himalayan Tradition, the Divine is also approached as Divine Mother.) Like the process described here, his method also is applied continually in ordinary daily routine and not just during special periods of practice. It is a living meditation achieved through developing a steady habit of alert and calm self-observation, which over time unfolds the Inner Witness and then the Centre of Consciousness. In the Himalayan Tradition the addition of initiation and the personal mantra become the foundations for the process.

> "It is necessary to lay stress on three things: (1) an entire quietness and calm of the mind and the whole being, (2) a continuance of the movement of purification ... (3) the maintenance in all conditions and through all experiences of the adoration and bhakti for the Mother."
> Sri Aurobindo, 1971, p887.

Thus through the grace of the Inner Teacher, the engine of initiation, and the discipline of meditation, the awareness of the Centre of Consciousness becomes stable, natural and spontaneous. What was just the faltering glimpse of the rising Sun of Spirit in the eastern sky at dawn now gradually becomes a fully effulgent Light. The awareness has become meditation in action; life has become a living meditation and all living has been raised to the level of meditation. For whether that inner Sun be expressed in inner space or also through the reflection of an outer master, they are one and the same. The path now is fully entered upon. Prepare to tread it, Oh disciple!

Direct Meditation on the Centre of Consciousness

Sit in your meditation posture with the head, neck and trunk straight. ...
    Let the body become steady, stable and absolutely still. ...

With a single, long exhalation, travel through body from head to toe and relax any tension in the muscle groups. ...
    Exhale any tension you find. ...

Let the breathing become diaphragmatic and connected, ...
    Quiet, ... deep, ... slow, ... smooth, ... equal ... and continuous. ...
    Let the whole body breath this way from top to toe and toe to top.

Now sense the energy field of the body. ...
    Feel the body's aliveness. ...
    This field is a gateway to the Inner Presence. ...
    Become one with, absorbed in that aliveness, the energy of that aliveness. ...

When your guru mantra appears just let it go, let it pulse continuously in the background as you relax and let it lead you deeper into stillness, into pure Silence. ...

A Silence that is absolutely still. ...
    A Silence that is a Conscious Presence; a Presence that can only be referred to as THAT. ...
    As though the whole of infinite inner space is alive, aware. ...
    As though the space in a room were pure awareness, pure conscious Presence, containing within it all the contents of the room and yet unaffected by their presence. ...
    Similarly the whole of inner space is pure Awareness, pure conscious Presence, containing within It all the contents of the mind and the ego, the small self, and yet remaining unaffected by them. ...
    A Nothingness, a Space, a Void of purest Awareness. ... Yet a Nothing that is Something. ...
    A Void that is a Plenitude; ... a Fullness of infinite potential. ...
    Recall the opening words of the *Isha Upanishad* :
        "That is full; this is full. This fullness has been projected from that fullness.
        When this fullness merges in that fullness, all that remains is fullness." ...

The power and presence of the eternal NOW. ...

That Presence may be effulgent with the softest white or golden light. ...
And if the mind is still enough you may detect a continual whispering: ...
> The whispering of a flow of purest knowing and certainty. ...
>> This is the Inner Teacher. ...
> The gentle caress of a downward flow of bliss. ...
>> This is the Inner Beloved. ... Love whispers. ...
You may even be aware of the subtle sounds in the right ear in the background. ...
> For some are led by sound and some by light. ...
Thoughts, images or feelings may flow through the inner space of the mind. ...
> Let them go like clouds scudding through the space of the sky. ...

The Presence becomes foreground; thoughts become only a distant murmuring background that no longer disturbs the Presence. ...
If there be even the slightest stirring of that silent Void, let it come forth as your mantra. ...
> Then refine it back into that Silence. ...
> Move back and forth between the pulsing of the mantra and the Silence as needed to stabilize the Presence. ...
Just be absorbed in THAT, ... in total Silence, ... in total Stillness, ... in total Awareness. ...
Rest in *Shanti*; ... in total Peace; ... in the "Peace that passes all understanding." ...

.....　　.....　　.....　　.....

Now let your mantra reappear. ....
Lead it gently and slowly towards the surface of the mind. ...
Join it with the breath, the two flowing together at the nostrils as though from a common point deep in the mind. ...
Maintaining the stillness and the mantra in the mind, gently cup the eyes with the palms of the hands. ...
Remaining inwardly attuned gently open the eyes to the palms, lower the hands to the thighs, move the body and be comfortable.

V THE BLESSING

The Opportunity

100. To come under the guidance of a Master is a blessing rare, and of the Inner Teacher, rarer still.

This sutra stresses the need for the student to have appropriate appreciation for the grace and blessings inherent in the opportunity provided by having both a Guru and a life supportive of spiritual endeavour and practice. Through this appreciation of the significance and rarity of this grace the student is encouraged not to waste a moment of this opportunity in frivolous worldly pursuits.

The importance of this opportunity is beautifully explained in a text by the Tibetan Buddhist master, Tsongkapa, who was born over six centuries ago. He wrote a text entitled the Source of All My Good which is presented with commentary in Preparing for Tantra: The Mountain of Blessings (Tsongkapa, 1995).

The text has four parts. The first is how to take a lama (i.e. a master in the Himalayan Tradition) and to serve him or her properly as the very root of the Path. The second is how to train your mind once you have taken a master. The third part is a request that you can attain all of the favourable conditions for succeeding on the Path, and to stop obstacles that might prevent you. Finally there is a prayer that in all future lives you may be taken under the care of a master, thereby gaining the strength to reach the final goal of enlightenment.

The importance of the master has been explored in sutras 68 to 75 above. From Tsongkapa's text:

> "The Buddha of Wisdom spoke to Tsongkapa, and said: "You must come to see that the Lama is one and the same with your high secret Angel, and pray to them - never stop praying, and then the seed which I have planted in you this day will flower, and you will understand all."

This brief excerpt makes the point that the master and the Centre of Consciousness are one and the same. It stresses the importance of initiation and the method of unceasing worship of the Centre.

101. Learn to take the essence of such a life.

In the second major part of this Tibetan text the advice is to take the essence of life:

> Bless me first to realize
> That the excellent life
> Of leisure I've found
> Just this once
> Is ever so hard to find
> And ever so valuable;
> Grant me then
> To wish, and never stop to wish,
> That I could take
> Its essence night and day."

If you are a serious and committed disciple there will come a time, a lifetime or a period within a lifetime when there is the opportunity to practice spirituality, to practice yoga. The outer conditions to succeed will be present. You will receive the grace of a master once major karmic duties have been discharged. There will be time to devote full attention to practice without significant distraction and supported by the availability of the necessary resources such as time, place, texts and teachings, funds, limited demands from relationships, etc. Inner conditions will also be present such as a healthy body and a mind that is endowed with the intelligence required to advance through the stages of the Path involving learning, contemplation and meditation. Spiritual advancement towards enlightenment both in this life and in the next (referred to as next life planning in the *vanaprastha* or forest dweller stage of the life cycle - retirement in the West), can be achieved because of the extraordinary kind of life one has now gained. When you are so blessed, you should seek to appreciate and truly recognize how significant this one opportunity really is.

Yet so many of us fail to work at our practice here and now in these special days of opportunity. We are bound by the habits and routines of everyday living and plunge ourselves into meaningless activities to gain material things, or other people's approval, or a taste of fame or power, or to entertain ourselves, or to fit into society's demands. We become so busy that we have in effect invented yet another way to lack spiritual opportunity. This is the challenge of renunciation for something higher than just everyday living. The force and momentum of habitual living is very powerful.

Eknath Easwaran stresses the importance of slowing down as part of his eight point program of meditation (Easwaran, 1978). Here we have a wonderful life of opportunity with a body and personality of exactly the same kind that

182 Sutras of the Inner Teacher

masters in the past have used to achieve enlightenment. Yet we use these things to collect bad deeds. Our spiritual leisure and fortune have been turned into a rich opportunity for suffering.

The gist of the verse is that we must take some special essence of these circumstances of opportunity so as not to lose these good qualities in future lives. We must use this lifetime, just this once, where everything has come together for us without a single essential piece of the whole incomplete. Otherwise we will lose this opportunity through lack of appreciation and it may be extremely difficult for us to find a life of spiritual leisure and fortune ever again. It is said that opportunity only knocks once. The good karma that created this life will be expended and wasted and will have to be rebuilt.

And so the verse is a request to our master that he or she bless us to achieve a commitment to the importance of this spiritual opportunity: *"bless me first to realize that the excellent life I've found,"* complete with every spiritual leisure, is hard to find and' - once found - is *"ever so valuable."* ... And *"grant me then to wish, and never stop to wish, that I could take this life's essence night and day:"* that I could at every given moment keep this precious time from being lost to actions which are pointless and devoid of any meaning." (Tsongkapa, 1995, p40-41).

The Essential Path

The sutras above have presented a complete and integrated practice of yoga, which we have chosen to call Samahita Yoga, which is suitable for this stage on the Spiritual Path. The final sutras summarize its essence.

102. The core practices for the Path are now five:

103. Act with unyielding integrity and discrimination through moral behaviour as guided by Spirit, as though death were looking over your shoulder.

104. Develop quietness, calmness, stillness, tranquillity and equanimity of mind, breath and body.

105. Purify the personality through worldly detachment and surrender to the Centre.

106. Develop a one-pointed mind.

107. In all conditions and through all experiences meditate with unceasing worship of the Centre of Consciousness.

108. But foremost is the grace of the Master, the Inner Teacher.

These Samahita sutras can be epitomized this way:

Follow your Centre without wavering!

OR

"Hold fast to That which has neither substance nor existence.
Listen only to the Voice which is soundless.
Look only on That which is invisible alike to the inner and outer sense."
Collins, 1976, p15

From us to you, dear reader, we offer our blessings:

*We bow our heads and join our hands before our hearts.
With all the power of thought in the mind,
With all the power of speech in the mouth,
With all the power of action in the hands,
We give you the blessings of the Himalayan Lineage and the Inner Teacher,
And worship the divinity, the Centre of Consciousness, within you.
Om shanti, shanti, shanti.
Peace, peace, peace
(Adapted from a blessing by Swami Veda Bharati)*

End Notes

1. The neurophysiology of emotion.

The subjective feelings we call emotions are an essential feature of normal human experience. Emotional purification is central to yoga *sadhana*. But what are emotions actually? The product or emergent property of our neurology? The result of our biochemistry - the so-called psychosomatic network? Or something more subtle as the experience of subtle energy fields in the *pranamayakosha* or *manomayakosha* of the subtle energy body - some even use the term "emotional body"?

At the level of neurophysiology emotions are expressed through physiological changes of the autonomic nervous system (ANS) and through stereotyped motor responses, especially of the facial muscles (Purves, 1997). The subjective experiences are much the same in all cultures.

Emotional expression is linked closely to the ANS through activity of certain brain stem nuclei, the hypothalamus and the amygdala, and structures in the spinal cord along with the autonomic ganglia. The limbic system refers to all of the centres that coordinate emotional responses.

Emotional arousal changes the activity of the sympathetic, parasympathetic and enteric (gastrointestinal) components of the ANS controlling cardiac and smooth muscle, and glands resulting in changes in sweating, heart rate, blood flow in the skin (blushing or pallor), piloerection (body hairs standing on end), and gastrointestinal mobility. This is tied into the "fight or flight" alarm mechanisms of stress. Different patterns of activation characterize various situations and their associated emotions. Various patterns of facial muscle activity are associated with specific patterns of ANS activity. Muscular expression of a particular emotion may lead to the subjective experience of that emotion.

The hypothalamus regulates many behaviours including body temperature, sexual activity and the endocrinology of reproduction. But in this regard it also regulates aggressive attack-and-defence behaviours, such as sham rage in cats. Indeed some researchers feel that emotional behaviours are often directed toward self-preservation - a point also made by Charles Darwin in his book on the evolution of emotion.

Papez (1937) suggested that the limbic lobe, originally part of the rhinencephalon (olfactory bulbs plus limbic structures) responsible for the sense of smell, was involved in emotional expression. The limbic lobe contains the cortex on the medial aspect of the cerebral hemisphere that forms a rim around the corpus callosum that connects both hemispheres together. It includes the cingulate gyrus and the hippocampus. He described a circuit in which the mammillary bodies of the hypothalamus project to the anterior nucleus of the dorsal thalamus and then to the cingulate cortex. It, in turn, projects to the hippocampus that then projects via a fibre bundle called the fornix back to the hypothalamus. These pathways underlie cortical control of emotional expression.

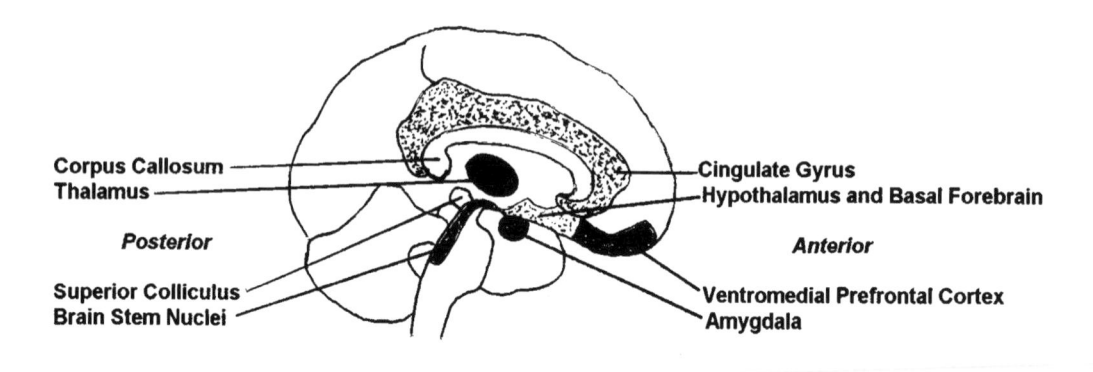

Key parts of the limbic system on the medial surface of the left side of the brain.

Paul MacLean (1984) extended this model of the limbic system with many more connections and the addition of the amygdala which connects extensively with the cerebral cortex and the hypothalamus. The amygdaloid complex is a critical link in the processes that give sensory experience their emotional significance. It evaluates and gives meaning to stimuli such as aversive conditioning of auditory stimuli in animals.

MacLean proposed a triune brain in which emotional processing depends upon an old mammalian brain or limbic system sandwiched between a more primitive, lower motor system called the reptilian brain, and a higher new mammalian system in the cerebral neocortex responsible for reasoning and thinking, all reciprocally interconnected. The reptilian system located at the core of the human brain controls unconscious stereotyped motor behaviours resembling the behaviour of reptiles, through the extrapyramidal motor system.

The limbic system has three functional subdivisions that regulate different emotional reactions. One controls the feelings and behaviours needed for self-preservation like feeding and fighting. A second regulates primal sexuality through feelings and behaviours that promote mating and copulation, and hence is concerned with species survival. These two subdivisions are connected to the reptilian brain via the medial forebrain bundle, and both project to the cingulate gyrus which is a primitive emotional cortex where such feelings can be experienced. The third subdivision links the cingulate gyrus with the hypothalamus to deal with feelings and behaviours that regulate maternal care and play. Thus the three subdivisions control emotions related to personal survival (first system), reproduction (second system) and survival of offspring (third system). Some investigators consider this concept of the limbic system as outmoded, but the idea remains in the absence of anything newer to replace it.

The two cerebral hemispheres contribute differently to the control of emotion. Damage to portions of the right hemisphere result in loss of ability to express emotion by modulation of speech patterns (aprosody). Such individuals cannot express emotion in speech but still have normal emotional feelings. The left hemisphere is more concerned with positive emotions and the right with negative emotions. The right hemisphere is involved in identifying emotions from facial expressions. Although both hemispheres participate, the right hemisphere overall is more involved in the perception and expression of emotions.

Studies of: 1) the effects of electrical or chemical stimulation of real brains; 2) the clinical effects of brain damage; and 3) recordings from the brains of people doing various tasks (so-called "wet cognitive science" since real brain experiments are involved), have led to the view that both the qualitative and quantitative aspects of the physical world seem to arise from evolved emergent properties of the nervous system rather than from events in the world that activate them. The colour yellow is not "out there". Lemons do not appear yellow because they really are yellow. Rather yellowness is an emergent property arising in the brain from the arrangements and interactions among the nerve cells that make up the neural networks of the brain. From this materialistic perspective feeling and consciousness are functional emergent properties of neural networks. Our sensory experience of the world is a grand illusion.

Evolutionary functionalism (Johnston, 1999) views emotions as the result of evolutionary forces. Over generations natural selection has created the neural machinery capable of producing emergent properties like emotions which have been favoured because they enhance reproduction and hence gene survival. The function of gene survival always dictates structural design. Feelings are not learned, but evolve by natural selection as emergent properties of the nervous system. Emotions have hedonic tone - the evaluative nature of a feeling, its pleasantness or unpleasantness. Positive or negative hedonic tone is closely related to whether the events that evoke it enhance or reduce the survival of our genes. Thus in evolutionary functionalism emotions are seen as "qualitatively different conscious states that have evolved to represent the nature, magnitude, and direction of expected threats or benefits to some aspect of our personal fitness." (Johnston, 1999, p86). The theory rests on data derived from computer simulations of the evolutionary process and on evidence for adaptive historical design.

Thus according to evolutionary functionalism our minds have evolved a library of emergent properties, including emotions, whose sole function has been the enhancement of our biological survival. As a theory of mind and emotions, evolutionary functionalism says that by favouring adaptive and functional emergent mental characteristics, natural selection has dictated the structure and organization of brains that are capable of exhibiting these properties. These are emergent properties evoked by those aspects of the physical and social world that are important for gene survival.

There is not universal agreement about what constitutes an emotion (Damasio, 1999). The six primary or universal emotions are happiness, sadness, fear, anger, surprise and disgust. Examples of secondary or social emotions are embarrassment, jealousy, guilt or pride. There are also background emotions like well-being, malaise, calm or tension, and the term has even been applied to feelings associated with drives, motivation and states of pain and pleasure. But all of these phenomena share a biological core of complicated patterns of chemical and neurological responses which play a regulatory role to create circumstances advantageous for survival of the organism. They are biologically determined processes arising from specific brain structures that have been laid down during a long evolutionary history - even though learning and culture can alter emotional expression and meaning. The neural substrates of emotion are triggered automatically leading to stereotypical responses with a regulatory purpose that have their effect on the body's internal milieu as well as on its visceral, vestibular and musculoskeletal systems.

At a biochemical level Pert (1997) sees emotions arising as a result of the operation of the psychosomatic network. The peptides that mediate the network make up a universal biochemical language of emotions whose influence extends throughout the organism rather than just within the brain. This chemical network integrates mental, emotional and biological activities (see end note 2 on psychoneuroimmunology and end note 5, p198, for additional details).

A completely different conception of emotions is held by psychic healers who work with the human aura and energy field. Many are sensitive and can sense thoughts and emotions in the human energy field as well as their movement between people in time and space (Brennan, 1987). Psychics describe a variety of models of the human energy field that include an emotional or astral body that forms as a layer in the subtle body or *pranamayakosha*. But there is little agreement on the nomenclature or the structure of these fields.

A recent and very different conceptualization of emotions comes from energy psychology (Gallo, 1999). It postulates that psychopathology and some physical symptoms can be treated through the subtle energy systems of the body. The cause of negative emotions and some physical symptoms is viewed as a disruption in the body's energy system. This is reminiscent of the yogic concept of localized turbulence, whirlpools or disruptions of the normally harmonious flow of the fields of prana in the subtle body (turbulent versus laminar flow in a fluid in physics). Energy psychology sees the essence of psychological problems as a disruption of the body's energy fields. This energetic disruption triggers and instructs all the rest of the physical processes that underlie emotional expression behaviourally, systemically, cognitively, neurologically and chemically. Remembering that we have said in the sutras that prana is the missing link between mind and body, this idea is potentially compatible with the more biological based descriptions reviewed above as an extension of the chain of causation. Clearly thought, emotion, sensation and physiology/biochemistry operate as an instantaneous unity, whatever the actual mechanisms may be.

If thoughts exist in fields (and in yoga the mind is conceived of as a very subtle energy field), and negative emotions consist as turbulent energy configurations, then psychological phenomena can be considered fundamentally as quantum mechanical events or processes, since quantum physics deals with the domain of subtle energy (Gallo, 1999). Since energy fields form with very low inertia, then psychological problems can be resolved easily by altering the energy field. At this point energy psychology is still too new, hardly even a discipline, to be able to evaluate these ideas. But the preliminary anecdotal clinical evidence of the rapidity, ease, power and permanence of these meridian interventions for relieving emotional and some functional physical problems is very impressive. These meridian therapies should be considered to be a practical extension of *prana vidya* in yoga and should be explored for their efficacy in easing the purification process of yogic *sadhana*.

2. Psychoneuroimmunology

Although many of the studies are old, three major lines of experimental evidence underlie the PNI hypothesis. The first correlates psychological factors with physiological effects.

PSYCHONEUROIMMUNOLOGY
Evidence

- Stress alters the functioning of both the immune and the neuroendocrine systems.
- Pavlovian conditioning (a form of learning) influences both the neuroendocrine and immune systems.
- The immune and nervous systems mutually affect and interact with each other. Cells of the immune system function in a sensory capacity to tell the brain about stimuli which would not be detected by the classical sensory system (invading foreign pathogens and cancer cells).

The second line of evidence is that Pavlovian conditioning as a type of learning influences the immune as well as the nervous system.

The third line of evidence documents the pervasive interlinks through which the nervous and immune systems influence each other. Both systems communicate mutually using immune, hormonal and neurotransmitters through interactions which are both anatomic and chemical.

Immune cells carry receptors for many neurotransmitters and hormones, and also secrete hormones and neurotransmitters as well as interleukins and immune mediators. Cells of the nervous, endocrine and immune systems share a pool of chemical mediators and receptors, including neurotransmitters, hormones and cytokines (immune mediators) to form what Pert (1997) has called a psychosomatic network that acts as a final common pathway for their joint functioning as an integrated multisystem network.

So the traditional hypothalamic/pituitary/adrenal axis now is known to have connections to the immune system to handle non-cognitive stimuli. There are regulatory feed back loops that link the nervous, the endocrine and the immune systems into a functioning unity. Environment and behaviour, in the sense of life style, can play key roles. The homeostatic nature of all these kinds of interactions is very important.

Both health and disease outcomes become a dynamic balance between pathogenic agents and processes on the one hand, and host resistance on the other. In other words, the seeds of disease require a fertile "soil" in which to flourish. PNI, or host resistance, refers to the quality of that "soil".

Now, the "soil" of host resistance is not just immunity, as is commonly thought. Imagine it to be more like a pie with many slices. And each slice has a different size in different contexts. There are slices for each of the components of the PNI system, for neuropeptides and growth factors, for nutrition and other factors, and likely for many other influences of which we are as yet unaware.

For the whole system the locus of control is at the plasma membranes, the surfaces of participating cells. Its essence is molecular communication between cell surfaces; the triggering of receptors by transmitters, cytokines and hormones to activate or suppress genes inside the participating cells. There is a continuous informational exchange within this internal cellular milieu.

3. Neurocardiology

The heart has its own independent nervous system called "the brain in the heart" that contains a complex network of at least 40,000 neurons - as many as are found in some subcortical brain centres (Childre and Martin, 1999). It used to be thought that the brain controlled the functioning of the heart by one-way signals via the sympathetic and parasympathetic nerves of the autonomic nervous system. But there is a two-way communication between the heart and the brain that projects to the amygdala, the thalamus and the cortex. These three structures work together to compare new information coming into the brain with memory for emotional significance (amygdala) and then decide what actions would be appropriate (cortex).

Sensory neurites in this network respond to stimuli such as blood pressure, heart rate, hormones and neurotransmitters. Several types of local circuit neurons arranged in processing stations integrate incoming nerve impulses from the brain and bodily organs with those coming from the heart's sensory neurites. This signal processing results in messages being sent from the heart to the medulla of the brain stem, and thence to higher centres, as well as to two pathways of the autonomic nervous system: sympathetic afferent (to the brain) nerves through the thoracic spinal cord and parasympathetic afferent nerves via the vagus nerve.

Besides this neurological communication the heart "talks" with the brain and the rest of the body biochemically (through hormones, especially atrial natriuretic factor produced by the heart, and neurotransmitters), biophysically (through pressure waves), and energetically (through electromagnetic field interactions). The research has shown that communication from the heart can influence brain function and a person's behaviour. Rhythmic beating patterns of the heart generate neural impulses that directly affect the electrical activity of the higher brain centres which mediate cognitive and emotional processing. (Note that the heart beat itself is generated from within the heart independent of the brain from the sino-atrial node as the dominant pace maker. Myocardial fibres have inherent rhythmicity.) The research further shows that positive emotions such as happiness, appreciation, compassion, care, and love reduce sympathetic (stress) stimulation of the heart and enhance parasympathetic activity (relaxation), as well as improving hormonal balance and immunity. They increase order and balance in the autonomic nervous system resulting in more efficient brain function.

Yogis are well familiar with how emotions alter breathing patterns. But emotional states are also reflected in heart rhythms as measured by heart rate variability (the beat to beat changes in heart rate). Since the heart is the strongest biological oscillator in the body, it entrains the other body systems with its own rhythm. The hypothesis is that:

> "As we perceive and react to the world, messages sent by the brain through the autonomic nervous system affect the heart's beating patterns. At the same time, the heart's rhythmic activity generates nerve signals that travel back to the brain, influencing our perceptions, mental processes, and feeling states."
> Childre & Martin, 1999, p26

Negative emotions like anger and frustration create disorder and incoherence in the heart's rhythm and in the autonomic nervous system, which then affect the rest of the body to create inefficient organ functioning and stress. Positive emotions do the opposite - enhanced harmony, order and coherence in the heart rhythm and balance in the nervous system. Thus heart rate variability, which reflects synchronization between the sympathetic and parasympathetic nervous systems, can be looked at as an indicator of mental and emotional balance, in the same way as alternate nostril dominance can be in *svara yoga*. Stress can create a disordered heart rhythm and subsequent effects like blood vessel constriction, a rise in blood pressure, and wasted energy.

The theory goes on to say that the "heart brain" is also the source of both positive (or heart) emotions (like compassion, etc.) as well as intuition. But the evidence is not supportive, any more than that the intestine is the source of the "gut feeling" of instinct. There appears to be a confusion of the heart as a physical organ with emotion, intuition, intellect and ego as functions of the mind. However, the interventions that have been devised by the HeartMath project based on this research are powerful anti-stress modalities, and can allow one to generate strong positive emotions like appreciation or gratitude consciously and at will. Some of them are reminiscent of Buddhist loving-kindness and heart meditations. The ability to generate high energy, positive emotional states at will is an important skill for the transpersonal visioning processes of Karma Yoga discussed in the sutras.

4. The Holographic Universe.

Brennan (1987) develops a holographic model out of Harmon's M-3 metaphysics. What is a hologram? In 1947 Gabor derived equations for holography as a kind of 3-dimensional photography (Talbot, 1991). In 1965 Leith and Upatinicks produced the first one using a laser. The process requires two steps. First the laser beam is split with a half beam splitter so that using reflecting mirrors half of the beam falls on the object (e.g. an apple) and the other half does not but acts as a reference beam. Both are reflected on to a photographic plate to interact with each other to produce an interference pattern. In the second step the hologram is projected by focussing a laser on the image of the interference pattern on the photographic plate with a lens. A 3-dimensional image of the object (e.g. the apple) appears suspended in space above the plate.

In a hologram, the part contains the whole; pieces of the photographic plate still project the whole apple, but the image is hazier since there is less information. Again the ancient wisdom describes the same idea: the microcosm (the human personality) contains the macrocosm (all the universal laws and principles); mastery of the part (the human personality) masters the whole: as above, so below.

In 1971, David Bohm, a student of Einstein, put forth the idea that the organization of the universe was probably holographic (Bohm, 1983). It consisted of implicate (like the interference pattern on the photographic plate) and explicate (like the suspended image of the apple) realities.

Soon thereafter, in trying to account for the puzzle of memory which seemed to be distributed all over the brain, probably as a field of energy, Karl Pribram at Stanford proposed that the human brain functions as a hologram, collecting and reading information from a holographic universe (Pribram, 1991).

194 Sutras of the Inner Teacher

Now Brennan (1987) advances a holographic model for energy healing that is based on seven premises about the nature of reality, which we paraphrase briefly here:

1. Consciousness is the basic reality. Karl Pribram has said that the senses create the illusion of a physical world (the apple) from universal energy fields around us (the interference pattern in the photographic plate). The basic reality is energy, not matter. This is M-3 metaphysics; consciousness is more fundamental. Thus any scientific or medical study based on the physical world, is a study of secondary and not primary causes.

2. Everything is connected to everything else. This is a premise consistent with general systems theory. There can be no observer, no independent parts. The scientific concept of a neutral and independent observer is a myth (Slife & Williams, 1995; Chalmers, 1982).

3. Each piece contains the whole. Each cell contains the full genome. At an energetic level, the energy field of each cell contains the pattern of the whole. Brennan now extrapolates these first three premises. All that there is, is in each of us. Heal yourself and you help heal others, the earth and the universe. As a part of the earth if you heal yourself then the earth is healed to that extent since you are a part of it This is the holographic principle according to Brennan.

4. Time is also holographic. Every aspect exists in all times and at all times. This is the eternal now of the meditative tradition. Meditation is a state of awareness characterized by thoughtlessness (mindlessness), timelessness and bliss/pure awareness/Silence. Thus time is no barrier to accessing resources in the transcendent world.

5. Individuation and energy are basic to the universe. From modern physics every aspect of the universe is either a wave of energy or an individual particle of energy. One might think of oneself as light, and not solid matter. This way one might be able to change more easily. Each second we have a different body. Each of us is unique, and what we experience is unique. The medical model treats everyone as the same (e.g. the clinical trial). We may allow for subgroups, but even within those subgroups there is a standard recipe for all.

6. The whole is greater than the sum of the parts. In the hologram, reconnect the pieces of the photographic plate and the image of the apple gets clearer. This is a model of systems within systems, with each having knowledge (awareness, consciousness) of all the others as one moves to successively higher and larger orders of organization. Bell's theorem in physics leading to the postulate of the conscious universe is relevant here (Kafatos & Nadeau, 1990). Summing the parts clarifies the whole. Teams and groups synergize. Brennan extrapolates these ideas to assert that we each have access to all the healing knowledge and power there is, ever was, and ever will be in the universe.

7. Consciousness creates reality and its own experience of reality. Karl Pribram

proposes that the brain processes data consistent with what it is used to (Pribram, 1991). One experiences according to one's expectations, which, in turn, are based on one's beliefs. This refers to the concepts of paradigms and models of the world explored in the sutras. Since reality is created by consciousness, it also creates its own experience of that reality, since that is also a part of that reality. This concept leads quickly to a big controversy in New Age thinking. For example, in the field of health, do we create our own disease, or just our own experience of it (suffering)? Do we create our own health? Are we responsible for our own suffering? Are we guilty? Are we bad? Brennan (1987) says that having responsibility for something does not mean being blamed for it (I'm ill because I've been bad). If we create our own experience of reality, we can also create something more desirable. The catch is, who does the creating? From what level of our being is this creating stemming? The central issue here is whether we create our own reality (implying there is no separate reality "out there"), or our <u>experience</u> of that reality (implying there is some kind of separate reality "out there" made up of fields and particles). We tend to the latter.

Brennan's holographic model with its seven premises is very speculative, and New Age, but it does reflect some of the understandings of modern quantum physics as well as the perennial wisdom.

5. The Scientific Study of Consciousness.

Let us review briefly some examples of the approach of Western science to the study of consciousness and contrast them with the Perennial Wisdom. The scientific study of spirituality is actually about the scientific study of consciousness.

What does Physics Say About Consciousness?

Classical physics has no place for consciousness. It has a local-reductionistic aspect. The sole ingredients of the physical universe are particles and local fields (forces). Every physical system is completely described by specifying the disposition in time and space of these two components. Its deterministic aspect shows that knowing the starting disposition of these components of a physical system, the laws of motion determine their disposition for all time. This implies that the motions of material things can be controlled only by the forces of classical physics which themselves are deterministically controlled. The system is logically complete. Conscious experience is superfluous. The evolution of the universe would be exactly the same whether subjective conscious experience exists or not. The issue is not whether conscious is real, but that it is not needed. It could only passively watch a preprogrammed course of events. But after three centuries we have failed to reconcile the properties of mind with the concepts of classical physics. Classical physical theory cannot provide an adequate conceptual foundation to understand mind-body (brain) dynamics.

But quantum theory can make a place for consciousness and there is considerable theoretical exploration taking place (Stapp, 1993; Goswamy, 1995; Tipler, 1994). Two key new concepts allow this change. Heisenberg's indeterminancy (uncertainty) principle in 1927 showed that it is impossible to know both the exact position and exact momentum for an object at the same time. We cannot know the future because we cannot know the present, except as possibilities. A mathematical theorem by Bell in 1964 that was proven experimentally in 1982 by Alain Aspect at the University of Paris-South, shows that physical reality in quantum theory is non-local. One would expect a one-to-one correspondence between physical theory and physical reality: that the theory is a way to see into the essence of reality. Thus one would expect that a physical event cannot simultaneously influence another event without some direct mediation like sending a signal (the principle of local causes). But experiment shows that non-locality is a fact of nature even though it seems to violate our everyday experience of reality as discrete (made up of individual objects) and causal. Rather, correlations between results hold even if the regions in space in which they are observed are too distant from one another to allow signals traveling at the speed of light to go between the two points in the time allowed. Non-locality allows us to infer (though not to prove) that the universe can be viewed as a conscious system (Kafatos & Nadeau, 1990). But Kafatos and Nadeau are quick to point out that this has nothing to do with eastern metaphysics as some respected physicists like Fritjof Capra and David Bohm claim.

> "...the majority of physicists tend not to be terribly impressed by these efforts. ...most physicists seem to be convinced that physics has nothing to do with metaphysics, and that any attempt to force a dialogue between the two can only result in dangerous and groundless speculation."
> Kafetos & Nadeau, 1990, p3

But physicists like Henry Stapp believe that we have introduced into physics physical events that are counterparts to concious events. His Heisenberg/James (H/J) model is a synthesis of William James' ideas about mind and consciousness with quantum theory according to Heisenberg (Stapp, 1993). In his Principles of Psychology (1890) James decribes the Consciousness of Self as follows:

> "... This me is an empirical aggregate of things objectively known. The I that knows them cannot itself be an aggregate. Neither for psychological purposes need it be considered to be an unchanging metaphysical entity like the Soul, or a principle like the pure Ego, viewed as "out of time". It is a Thought, at each

moment different from that of the last moment, but appropriative of the latter, together with all that the latter called its own ... thought is itself the thinker, and psychology need not look beyond."

Thus for James, consciousness is just a thought: the witness of thought is just another thought. Mind suffices, it is all psychology. Stapp's H/J model uses this Jamesian mind which involves no "knower" that stands behind the thoughts themselves, and hence the model is less susceptible to Gilbert Ryle's influential description of the error of infinite regress, his ghost-in-the-machine.

In the H/J model reality is described by a probability distribution for the particle (Schrödinger's wave function). With detection, the wave function is said to "collapse" and a specific "detection event" is observed with a particular probability. By virtue of an act of detection or measurement by an observer, a general probability becomes a specific actuality. In this way the observer is said to influence the event. In H/J theory the brain is the measuring device and the observer is consciousness (i.e. mind - the feel of the actual brain quantum event).

Goswami (1995) says that it is the nonlocal consciousness that collapses the mind's wave function and then experiences the outcome of this collapse. Objects move from a transcendent possibility domain into a domain of manifestation when nonlocal, unitive consciousness (the experiencer or subject) collapses their wave functions. This collapse occurs in the presence of the awareness of a brain-mind as the measuring device.

> "Before the collapse, the state of the brain-mind thus exists as potentialities of myriad possible patterns that Heisenberg called tendencies. The collapse actualizes one of these tendencies, which leads to a conscious experience (with awareness) upon completion of the awareness. Importantly, the result of the measurement is a discontinuous event in space-time. ... consciousness chooses the outcome of the collapse of any and all quantum systems."
> Gosawami, 1995, p173.

As interesting as these models are, they deal only with how consciousness might interact with mind and matter. But they do not address the existence or nature of consciousness itself.

In acknowledging our ignorance about how consciousness interacts with the physical world, R.G. Jahn and B.J. Dunne at Princeton (quoted in Stapp, 1993) say:

> "The literature of physics research abounds with attempts to transpose various physical formalisms [to account for these effects]: electromagnetic models, thermodynamic models, mechanical models, statistical mechanical models,

hyperspace models, quantum mechanical models, and others ... Although these comprise an interesting body of effort, none of them seems fully competent. ... Indeed, it appears that no single application of existing physical theory is likely to prevail. In order to encompass the observed effects, a substantially more fundamental level of theoretical model will need to be deployed, one which more explicitly acknowledges the role of consciousness in the definition of physical reality."

What Does the Mind-Body Paradigm Say About Consciousness?

The Psychosomatic Network. Even the psychoneuroimmune (PNI) system is being examined by some scientists for its potential to be conscious. Pert (1997) refers to the PNI system as a single psychosomatic network which is drawn together by a set of informational molecules. These peptides act as the molecular messengers that facilitate the conversation among the nervous, endocrine and immune systems. These peptides are the hormones, neurotransmitters, endorphins, growth factors, cytokines, interleukins and other factors that mediate the activities of the PNI system and were originally studied in other contexts and known by other names. After many years it was recognized that they are a single family of molecular messengers which act by attaching themselves to the abundant specific receptors on the surfaces of all body cells like a key into a lock. By interlinking immune, endocrine and brain cells in this way these peptides form a psychosomatic network that extends throughout the entire organism to coordinate mental, emotional and biological (immune and endocrine) activities. Virtually every known peptide recognizes receptors on and is produced by all the constituent cells of the PNI system. Indeed it is now thought that traditional synaptic transmission in nerve cells is limited mainly to muscle contraction. Most of the signals from the brain and nervous system are transmitted via peptides emitted from nerve cells which can act throughout the whole body through the psychosomatic network. Pert's research suggests that AIDS may be rooted in a disruption of peptide communication since the HIV virus enters cells through particular peptide receptors.

Pert has hypothesized that the entire group of sixty or seventy peptides may constitute a universal biochemical language of emotions. Emotions are associated particularly with the limbic system of the brain which is highly enriched with peptides and their receptors, as is the intestinal tract ("gut feelings"). Most of these peptides alter mood and behavior. It is hypothesized that each peptide may evoke a particular emotional tone. The nervous pathways with their ganglia and nuclei that connect the sensory organs with the brain and act to filter and prioritize sensory perceptions, are enriched with peptide receptors. Thus all sensory perceptions, thoughts and bodily functions would be emotionally colored because they all involve peptides - which is our common experience. Unlike the central nervous system, a network is not hierarchically structured. As we will discuss below, this may imply that the phenomenon of cognition, of knowing, extends throughout the whole organism through this intricate chemical "psychosomatic network" of peptide informational molecules that integrates mental, emotional and biological activities.

> "The body is the unconscious mind" p141
> "If we accept the idea that peptides and other informational substances are the biochemicals of emotion, their distribution in the body's nerves has all kinds of significance, which Sigmund Freud, were he alive today, would gleefully point out as the molecular conformation of his theories." p141
> "...these biochemicals are the physiological substrates of emotion, the molecular underpinnings of what we experience as feelings, sensations, thoughts, drives, perhaps even spirit or soul." p130
> "I'd say that the fact that memory is encoded or stored at the receptor level means that memory processes are emotion-driven and unconscious." p143
> "Information theory seems to be converging with Eastern philosophy to suggest that the mind, the consciousness, consisting of information, exists first, prior to the "physical realm", which is secondary, merely an out-picturing of consciousness." p257
> Pert (1997)

Pert provides a telling little story of how Depak Chopra tried to explain to some rishis in India about her work on how neuropeptides and receptors communicate as informational molecules (Pert, 1997, p260). "But they could only shake their heads and give him a very quizzical look. Finally, the oldest and wisest appeared to suddenly get it. He sat straight up and with an expression of great surprise, said, 'Oh, I understand! She thinks these molecules are real!'"

Information Transduction. Rossi (1993, p131) has developed this information paradigm further claiming that "information theory is capable of unifying psychological, biological and physical phenomena into a single conceptual framework that can account for mind-body healing, personality development, the evolution of human consciousness, and a fascinating panorama of cultural practices"! He sees the basic laws of biology, psychology and cultural anthropology as essentially descriptions of different levels of information transduction.

His approach is based on Mishkin's psychobiological theory which is a synthesis of behaviorist and cognitive frameworks for understanding how memory and learning occur and the role of thinking, awareness and consciousness in the process. The first is behaviorism. Habits as automatic stimulus-response connections are formed whenever there is adequate reward as a basic process at all levels of life. The second is cognitive psychology. The evolution of the cortico-limbic-thalamic pathways in mammals allows the acquisition of information and knowledge plus a self-conscious and self-driven memory system.

He postulates that through mind-gene connections the informational molecules of the PNI system not only mediate mind-body communication, but also a type of mind-body encoding called state-dependent memory, learning and behavior (SDMLB) which he considers to be the hidden denominator behind most schools of psychotherapy ranging from hypnosis, psychoanalysis and behavior therapy to methods like imagery, relaxation and meditation. These state-dependent processes are encoded in the limbic-hypothalamic system and the related PNI system as the major centre of mind-body information transduction. Enduring psychosomatic symptoms are examples of experiential learning in response to stress in the form of state-bound response patterns of learning that are encoded within the limbic-hypothalamic-PNI system "filter" which modulates mind-body communication.

Rossi sees mind-body healing, therapeutic hypnosis, the placebo response and traditional practices of psychotherapy and holistic medicine as psychobiological processes of accessing and using SDMLB systems that encode symptoms and problems and then reframing them for improved adaptation, integration and personal development. He includes the ultradian rhythms of nostril dominance as part of the PNI system and refers to them as the "wave nature of consciousness" or the "Unification Hypothesis of Chronobiology".

He goes on to equate consciousness with mind and to define them as "a process of self-reflective information transduction mediated by the messenger molecules of the body" (ibid p10). But he does not discuss what this actually means.

The Relaxation Response. Readers will already be familiar with Herbert Benson's pioneering studies of the physiological responses to transcendental meditation (Benson et al, 1974), which he eventually formulated into the relaxation response. We now know that the PNI system mediates this response. But to characterize meditation as only the relaxation response is to trivialize it.

These few contemporary examples from psychobiology are instructive for showing the tendency to confuse mind and emotions with consciousness. There is an underlying materialistic assumption that mind and consciousness are composed of information (whatever that means) and are emergent properties of biochemistry - the peptides of the PNI system. This is a new twist on the human being as machine. At its basis our awareness, even our self-awareness, is purely chemistry. After being relegated for so long to a soft science, now psychology can at last find legitimacy in the hard sciences of physics and chemistry. It should be noted that we will return to this discussion below when we consider consciousness as an emergent property of self-organizing systems in cognitivism and Santiago Theory. The immune system is such a cognitive system.

What does Neuroscience say about Consciousness?

Precious little! Leaving cognitive science aside for the moment, a perusal of two current texts show only three paragraphs in a box on consciousness in one (Purves et al, 1997), and a two page appendix on psychomotor aspects of the brain-mind problem in the other (Henatsch, 1996). The study of psychomotor functions like intention, planning, recognition, comparison and other aspects of our doing, much less memory and learning, all contain mental elements. The relationship between physical and mental events is at the centre of the Cartesian brain-mind problem. There are some dualists who assert that the differences between brain and mental processes are so essential that they cannot be unified. But most neuroscientists follow monism that accepts only one elementary substance for both living and nonliving matter. Most modern monists are materialists - mental phenomena arise from and obey the same physico-chemical laws as the entire realm of nature. The physiology of sleep and wakefulness and the role of the reticular activating system and its neural connections that mediate them are dealt with at length in neuroscience. But despite great interest the definition of consciousness is uncertain, much less its evolutionary origin and relationship to the mechanics of brain function.

At one extreme scientists in the field of *artificial intelligence* think of brains as glorified computers. They argue in the extreme that any feedback device has the essential quality that would eventually lead to human consciousness. At the other extreme are arguments that only human beings are conscious. That because its operation in some ways resemble mental processes, therefore, a computer can be conscious has been refuted by Searl, who emphasizes that meaningful output from a computer, however sophisticated, can never provide evidence that it is conscious (Purves et al, 1997).

Two major challenges are freedom of will and action, and also self-consciousness, the internal observer or self. Not only do we know, but we know that we know, and have a sense of personal self as the knower. Yet no amount of analysis or examination can find an actual inner self. Despite centuries of debate the riddle remains unresolved. Neurobiologists now treat consciousness as an emergent property of the brain rather than as some kind of specific entity that can be studied in its own right. By *emergence* is meant the sudden appearance of previously unknown properties in a system. In the case of the brain it results from a long evolution towards ever more complex networks of neurons improving the chances of survival for the organism. The identity hypothesis eliminates mind by making it an emergent property of physico-chemical processes in the brain. A philosophical analysis called *neurophilosophy* has been developed to make a unified science of the mind-brain formulated in terms of cybernetic theory and neurophysiological data (Churchland,1986).

There is a *holistic theory* of thoughts (Guyton & Hall, 1996) formulated in terms of neural activity as a pattern of stimulation of many parts of the nervous system at the same time and in definite sequence, probably involving most importantly the cerebral cortex, thalamus, limbic system and upper reticular formation of the brain stem. Those areas of the limbic system, thalamus and reticular formation determine a thought's general nature (pleasant, unpleasant, gross sensory modality, body location, etc.). The cerebral cortex then determines finer characteristics of the five-sensory experience. Consciousness is then described as our continuing stream of awareness of both our surroundings and also our sequential thoughts.

Creutzfeld described an essential dilemma in any brain-mind research (Henatsch, 1996). Man converts the world experience by the senses into symbols of that reality in the form of language. These symbols are not the real world, but rather models of it described in mental constructs (the concept of paradigms or models of the world). The world as experienced and the model description belong to different philosophical categories. Thus any attempt to equate particular mental experiences with a specific brain mechanism compares "apples to oranges" and must ultimately fail.

Cognitive Science : Bringing Forth a World

Cognitive science refers to the study of the mind or what is *cognition*. It asks how we acquire, process, retain and use knowledge as a basis for action or to generate more knowledge. One way to study these phenomena is called "dry cognitive science" (DCS) which builds computer models of cognitive processes like decision making, and compares them to actual human behaviour. The other strategy called "wet cognitive science" (WCS), relies on real brain experiments and the study of neural networks. Artificial intelligence with its computer model of the mind dominates the field, but other disciplines are involved such as linguistics, neuroscience, psychology, sometimes anthropology, and the philosophy of mind. Its core is *cognitivism* with its guiding metaphor of the digital computer (DCS). Human cognition is the manipulation of symbols as in a digital computer. Cognition is the mental representation that results when the mind is thought to operate by manipulating symbols that represent the world in some way.

In opposition to this idea of cognition as mental representation and symbol processing as its vehicle, is the field of *connectionism* (WCS). It views cognitive tasks like vision or memory as global behaviors that emerge from neural networks (which are examples of systems made up of many simple components - neurons -that are connected by appropriate rules), which give rise to global behavior. Connectionist models substitute localized, symbolic processing for distributed operations extending over the entire network of components resulting in the emergence of new global properties that are resilient to malfunction. The representation is the correspondence between the emergent global state and the properties of the world. No preprogrammed processing of symbols is involved. The ability of neural networks to learn and to recognize patterns is an example.

A third and more recent stream of thought has been called *"enactive"* (Varela et al, 1991). It criticizes not only the idea of symbolic processing, but even that cognition is representation. Rather than thinking of cognition as the representation of a pre-given world by a pre-given mind as well as a subject who does it, cognition becomes an ongoing enactment of a world and a mind based on the history of the various actions that the being in the world performs. Cognition or knowing becomes a process of bringing forth rather than representing a world. One could consider it a further development of the concept of paradigms and models of the world discussed in the sutras.

The most influential version of the enactive model is the Santiago Theory of Cognition developed by Humberto Maturana and Francisco Varela about 1960. The essence of the theory is that mind is a process rather than a thing. Its central insight is that cognition, the process of knowing, is identical to the very process of life itself, including perception, emotions and behavior. As a process of knowing, cognition is much more than thinking. It is any perception or process of knowing about a change in the internal or external environment. It could be any perception, emotion, action, language or concept - even consciousness.

Mind and matter are considered as two different aspects of life, not as separate categories. The Cartesian split of mind, "the thinking thing" (*res cogitans*) and body (*res extensa*), is abandoned. Indeed one need not have a brain for a mind to exist, for by this definition cognition is a property of bacteria or plants that respond to and, therefore, perceive environmental change. The process of cognition operates through the entire structure of the organism, whether or not it has a brain and central nervous system. Mind is to brain as process is to structure. Mind is a process of cognition (rather than a thing that cognizes or knows) and brain is a specific structure through which mental process (the process of cognition or knowing) operates.

This mental process or cognition involves neither a transfer of information nor mental representations of the outside world. As a contemporary, Gregory Bateson presented similar ideas from cybernetics and systems theory, speaking in terms of patterns and relationships as the essence of nature and the living world (Capra, 1996). For Bateson, pattern, structure and process were the three key criteria of life. For him also, cognition as the process of knowing was the process of life. Biological form consists of relationships rather than parts. An organism like a fly could change (go through the process) - could grow, mature and senesce. But despite these structural changes its pattern retains its identity as an organism, as a fly, throughout.

Similarly Maturana and Varela view all living systems as autonomous networks that they describe as *autopoietic* (self-making, self-organizing) (Maturana & Varela, 1980; Maturana & Varela, 1998; Varela et al, 1991). They have a basic *circular organization* (somewhat analogous to feedback in systems) that makes them self-organizing; that is, components produce and transform other components (biochemical pathways, for example), to create continual structural change while preserving the web-like organizational pattern or identity of the system - much like the analogy of the fly above in Bateson's model. In this way the living system develops over time in a process of self-renewal arising from this cyclical structural change. These developmental structural changes create new structures in response to either environmental influences or to the internal dynamics of the system. Bateson saw a unity of mind and life, of mind and nature. And Maturana and Varela similarly have developed a new synthesis of mind, matter and life based on the interdependence of process, pattern and structure.

Key to this developmental process and its associated structural change in a living system is the role of the environment. A living system interacts with its environment through what Maturana and Varela call *structural coupling*. This describes recurrent interactions between the components of the living system (especially at its boundaries), and the components of the environment that trigger structural changes in the system. The environment only triggers the changes, but does not specify or direct them. The living system responds rather than reacts to its environment. If you kick a ball it reacts in a predictable way. If you kick a dog it will respond unpredictably, depending on its structure and developmental history. Thus a structurally coupled system is a learning system. In response to its environment, then, a living system adapts continually (and thereby exhibits learning), and undergoes continual structural changes.

Moreover, Maturana and Varela see living systems as *self-referring*. By this they mean that the processes of perception and cognition do not represent or even construct the pre-given, existing, external reality or world. Rather they specify one, "bring forth a world" through the process of circular organization in the nervous system that continually creates new relationships (structural change) within its neural network. (This is another way to talk about the uniqueness of what we call models of the world.) Maturana and Varela believe that this process of circular organization itself - with or without a nervous system - is identical to the process of cognition. "Living systems are cognitive systems, and living as a process is a process of cognition." (Maturana & Varela, 1998).

Cognitive Immunology

Santiago Theory has influenced many fields of science. One of these is immunology. Returning to the psychoneuroimmunne (PNI) system discussed in end note 2, Santiago Theory views the immune system as an autonomous, cognitive, self-organizing and self-regulating network that maintains the body's molecular identity. Varela and Coutinho (1991) propose that it does so by regulating an organism's cellular and molecular repertoire through structural coupling to its environment. The immune system has become the immune network. A war model of soldiers searching out to destroy an invading enemy is replaced by a communication network of people talking to each other.

Foreign molecules in minute amounts are incorporated naturally into ongoing regulatory activities of the immune network. The cognitive activity of the immune network results from its structural coupling to its environment, implying that these foreign molecules from the environment perturb the immune network, triggering structural changes in it that result in regulating their levels within the context of the system's other regulatory activities. Even though they are foreign, these molecules are not automatically destroyed.

However, when there is a massive invasion (eg. infection) that overwhelms and cannot be incorporated into the regulatory network of the immune system, then a massive defensive reaction typical of the immune response is triggered.

Varela sees autoimmunity as perhaps a failure in the cognitive operation of the immune network, which should be reinforced by boosting its connectivity. He also believes that any sophisticated psychosomatic or mind-body view of health requires conceptualizing the nervous and immune systems (i.e. the PNI system) as interacting cognitive systems - many "brains" in continuous conversation. By adding cognition (an ability to know) as a property of the PNI system, Santiago Theory provides an interesting dimension to the psychosomatic and informational network proposals of Pert and Rossi respectively as reviewed above.

Consciousness in Santiago Theory: Knowing that we Know

Consciousness in Santiago theory refers to the *self-awareness* that begins only in higher animals and manifests fully in the human mind (Varela et al, 1991). If cognition means knowing, then awareness of the environment is a property of cognition at all levels of life. To be conscious is to be aware not only of our environment but also of our inner world and ourselves. We know that we know. We are aware that we are aware.

In Santiago Theory self-awareness arises out of language that is studied through analysis of communication. Rather than a transmission of information as is commonly understood, here communication becomes how behaviour is coordinated among living organisms through mutual structural coupling (through recurrent mutual interactions). This distinction between coordination of behavior and information exchange (exchange of meaning) is key to the concept of communication in Santiago Theory. The distinction lies with this concept of structural coupling that arises from Varela's work with cellular automata- very simple computer experiments that show the emergence of regular (structural) behaviour when the components interact among themselves or their environment according to very simple pre-given rules (i.e. rules determined by their structure) (Varela et al, 1991). One could argue that peptide-receptor interactions in the psychosomatic network could be considered structural coupling, although biochemical, because of their "lock and key" conformational nature. Each interaction results in a predictable outcome or "behaviour" determined by the structure and connections of the receptors. Thus these structural interactions (couplings) coordinate the cellular behaviour in the psychosomatic network.

This seems a rather mechanical process compared to the formulation by Rossi or Pert in terms of information transduction and informational molecules respectively. Moreover, to view the response of an organism to its environment through this process of structural coupling as a behaviour that results from cognition or knowing (especially when the transfer of information is denied), and then to extend the concept that this cognition implies awareness of the environment seems to push and distort the usual meanings of these English words much too far with resulting confusion. To know and to be aware implies consciousness. To imply then that consciousness is simply an emergent property of this kind of mechanical or chemical structural coupling within a network, however complex, can be no more than pure conjecture. It would be very difficult indeed to prove the emergence of something like awareness or consciousness from a neural network.

Nevertheless, be that as it may, Santiago Theory ties the emergence of self-awareness closely to language. Maturana and Varela look at language also as a network of structural couplings or relationships among its words, concepts and abstractions (Varela et al, 1991; Maturana & Varela, 1998). Thus meaning is an emergent property of this pattern of relationships among linguistic distinctions just as other global properties emerge out of similar networks of densely interconnected components. Thus we come to exist in a "*semantic domain*" (what we call a model of the world - encoded in language), which emerges from the process of "*human languaging*". To be human is to weave continually this linguistic network in which we are embedded. To be human is to exist in language and the meaning that is emergent from it. In language we coordinate our behaviour and together in language we bring forth our world. "The world everyone sees is not <u>the</u> world but <u>a</u> world", which we bring forth with others." (Maturana & Varela, 1998). But the theory goes further. Self-awareness arises when we use "*languaging*" (abstract concepts and notions of objects) to describe ourselves. This semantic domain then expands in human beings to include reflection (self-awareness).

Varela calls this the "Cartesian anxiety" (Varela et al, 1991). The origins of this dilemma lie in our tendency to create abstractions of separate objects. That includes a separate self. And then having separated objects in this abstract way we come to believe they actually belong to an objective independently existing reality. To overcome this Cartesian anxiety Varela feels we need to think systemically about relationships rather than objects and to recognize that identity and individual autonomy do not imply separateness and independence. Varela's attraction to Buddhism goes beyond just the use of mindfulness meditation as an experiential and experimental method. The Buddhist doctrine of impermanence also includes the idea that there is no self. There is no persistent subject of all of our varying experiences. The idea of a separate or individual self is an illusion, just another form of *maya*, an intellectual concept that has no reality. For the Buddhist, clinging to this idea of a separate self leads to pain and suffering.

6. Consciousness in Advaita Vedanta

There are some six major schools of classical orthodox Indian philosophy (Indich, 1995). Each is called a *darshana* which comes from the verb *drsh* meaning "to see". The word darshana implies a vision of truth; a direct, immediate, intuitive or direct apperception or insight into the nature of Reality. Although a philosophy may be constructed around this vision, the vision itself is directly revealed. Among these major schools of philosophy the preeminent role is given to *Vedanta*. The word implies the culmination of the history and philosophy of Vedic or revealed wisdom. It has many versions, but *Advaitic* or *nondualistic Vedanta* as formulated by Shankara (788 - 820 AD) is key.

The basic claim of Vedanta is that transcendental, non-dual Consciousness is the essence of both the subjective and objective elements of our experience and of ultimate Reality Itself. This is a vision of a non-dual, transcendental and purely spiritual Reality. That Reality is called *Brahman* (God) or at the individual level *Atman* (soul). This is what constitutes the spiritual centre of the Vedantic model of the personality in figure 2. This concept of the Self underlies the essence of the understanding of the meaning of human life and of the nature of the universe that is called enlightenment. The science of yoga deals with the problem of pain and the process of its elimination as enlightenment is reached. Vedanta describes what that experience reveals to one who Knows. Note that this is basically an experiential statement, even though it has been elaborated into a philosophy.

Shankara used three sets of traditional texts to provide an authoritative scriptural basis for his vision. These texts are called the triple foundation of Vedanta, and are made up by the Upanishads, the Bhagavad Gita, and the Vedanta or Brahma Sutras. These are revealed texts, the record of the transcendental experiences of the sages in *samadhi*. They are not the product of the mind, *pramana*, which includes perception, inference and authority. While these latter can lead to truth, they can also lead to error. It is in these that our own Western science is grounded. In this philosophy the goal of life, mankind's highest goal, is to realize this ultimate Reality. It is to answer the question, "Who am I?".

Three statements lie at the heart of Advaita. The first is that Brahman or absolute Consciousness is non-dual and is unchanging Reality. The second is that the world is illusion (*maya*). And thirdly, man's Eternal Self (the Atman or Soul at the centre of the model of the personality in figure 2) is not different from that Reality or Brahman. Thus the central principle in Advaita Vedanta is the non-duality of Brahman, absolute Consciousness or Reality.

What is this Reality called Brahman? The Advaitic vision of Reality is summarized in the word, *saccidananda*. It is made up of three words. *Sat* means existence, truth or reality. *Cit* means consciousness, wisdom, or transcendental knowledge (in the sense of knowing), omniscience. *Ananda* refers to bliss and love. These should not be considered attributes of Brahman but rather that Brahman is these things. They are described as *svarupa*, of Its unitary essential nature. This Reality is the ground of all creation. To an embodied physical mind this absolute Consciousness or Brahman is unthinkable and indescribable, in other words, transcendent. Thus it is described by the *via negativa* embodied in the two words, *neti, neti* - "not this, not that".

What then is the world? This question is approached through two concepts. The first is *maya* and the second involves the distinction of *levels and degrees of reality*.

Maya is the power by which this absolute Consciousness or Brahman is concealed, and by which a distortion in the form of the apparent or manifested world occurs. Brahman with Its creative power *maya* is personified as *Ishvara*, the Lord, whose creation is the phenomenal world as His *lila* or play - a joyous, sportive, spontaneous activity of creation. This absolute Consciousness is eternally and spontaneously creative. To those who are involved in the relative world this phenomenal experience is real enough. But for those who Know, the experience of this absolute Consciousness is much more real, and relatively speaking the phenomenal world seems like a dream. Indeed the phenomenal world appears to emerge from absolute Consciousness or Brahman, but only when viewed from the context of the world itself. When viewed from the standpoint of absolute consciousness there is no world. This plurality, consciousness-with-an-object or subject-object consciousness is but an appearance. Actual reality is Consciousness-without-an-object, utter non-duality.

7. Subpersonalities

The concept of "parts" of the personality can be found in the number of psychotherapeutic systems, for example, Gestalt therapy, ego-state psychology and psychoanalysis. The concept has been particularly well developed in Neuro-Linguistic Programming. Swami Rama also refers to the concept in his commentary on the method of 61 points as a part of *yoga nidra* (Swami Rama, 1982a).

The origins of human behaviour can be thought of as consisting of various parts. This is an operational concept - a model - that looks at the mind functionally as though it were particulate or discontinuous. All of us have functional parts that do various normal activities. We have parts that can drive a car, parts that help us walk, etc. We also have parts operative in the unconscious mind that are responsible for physical and psychological symptoms and diseases. There are also parts that represent the functioning of bodily organs. One could imagine these as unique configurations of energy that lie in the mind and pranic fields. Since parts are suffused with consciousness, then they behave as though they were little people inside the personality, and one can communicate with them. When we talk popularly about the "inner healer" or my "inner child", we refer to a similar idea.

Using light hypnotic trance, with or without ideodynamic signalling (Rossi and Cheek, 1988) or by using muscle testing with kinesiology (Gallo, 1999), one can learn to communicate and work with parts to alter their functioning within the human personality overall. Changing the functioning of a part will result in a change in behaviour, both external behaviour and also internal behaviours such as internal states like feelings and emotions and bodily functioning. Feelings of resistance, for example, can interfere with the total commitment that is required to work with the Centre of Consciousness with integrity. The parts responsible for these feelings of resistance can be accessed. Often one finds more than one part (called aspects of the problem of resistance), and they may be in conflict about what is wanted. There are effective methods for achieving psychological integration of conflicting parts. Successful integration results in disappearance of the feelings of resistance and a full commitment to whatever action is contemplated.

A related phenomenon is a part that acts as an objector to any planned action or alteration in psychological structure. There are methods to reframe objectors so that they support committed and aligned action.

Finally, there are methods that can align all of the parts of the personality to the Centre of Consciousness leading to committed action with integrity.

8. Death

Signs of Immanent Death

In yoga philosophy our individual personal cycles of life and death are considered to be part of the larger cosmic cycles. The subtle body is the repository of those cosmic forces within the individual. Within each of us there is a link between personal and cosmic cycles. Indeed we saw an example above in the discussion of the cycles of the *svara* which is linked to the lunar cycles (sutra 20). These representatives of the cosmic forces within the subtle body are also affected through our karma. In other words, this same subtle body is also the repository of our *samskaras* which create karma. *Samskaras* represent the sum total of all the impressions of our thoughts, actions and experiences, however subliminal, stored in the unconscious mind. So when the rhythms of the cosmic forces are acted upon by our karmic residues in the causal body, they produce our diseases and our health; they determine our mode and moment of death; and they direct us to the next incarnation. They also warn us of impending death by producing varying types of symptoms.

The texts have many examples of signs of immanent death acting over minutes, hours, days, weeks or months prior. The Charaka Samhita, one of the most ancient medical texts in the world and a key text of Ayurvedic medicine, devotes chapters 5 to 11 of section V on the prognosis of death through fantasy, dreams and physiological signs. In the last chapter it discusses the signs of natural imbalances which cause medicines to become ineffective in the body. The *Shiva Svarodya* mentioned in sutra 20, one of the major texts on the science of breath rhythms or *svara*, devotes verses 321 to 369 to describing the symptoms that indicate impending death within a period of one year to the immediate future. Here are some sutras from the Markandeya and Skanda Puranas as further examples. The first two revisit *svara* and breath rhythms.

> "If only the left or only the right nostril is active for many days.
> If both nostrils are equally active for ten days (sushumna)."

There are some that make a little sense from the Western perspective:

> "One has consistent incontinence of bowl, bladder and ejaculation.
> One's intellectual processes become confused.
> One articulates different from what he intends.
> A fat person suddenly becomes lean or vice versa.
> One remains hungry even after a very full meal.

> One has a sudden and complete change of character: from
> gentle to violent or vices versa; a miser gives away all of
> his wealth or a generous person becomes miserly."

Many verses describe dreams that may indicate a short life span or impending death. For example, a series of texts deal with the *chayapurusha* or shadow man: the gigantic shadow figure one sees against a clear sky after gazing at one's shadow in sunlight or moonlight. Various signs in the shadow man of the sky can indicate impending death or a short remaining life span. Then there are others which seem strange to the Western mind:

> "One sees colours reversed (eg red for green).
> Tastes as reversed (eg bitter for sweet).
> One does not see his own shadow.
> One sees two moons or two suns.
> One sees the moon and the stars in the day.
> One sees no stars at night.
> One sees the sun or the moon but no rays thereof."

With reference to the latter let one of us relate an experience I had with my father. On two occasions he casually remarked on the beauty of two moons in the evening sky as though it were a perfectly ordinary thing. He was 85 years of age at the time, in apparent good health. He did not have diplopia and knew nothing of yoga. He died peacefully three months later exactly as predicted in the texts, and we were thereby prepared for it.

The psychic causes behind these experiences and phenomena are fully understood only by the yogis by reference to the factors in the subtle body, the inner of the five sheaths of the personality and their mutual interactions as described in Vedanta (sutra 16). It is mastery over these that leads to the conquest of death in the yoga science.

Types of Death

To the Westerner this is a peculiar one. After all, death is death, is it not? Not so in the Perennial Wisdom! It recognizes several kinds (Arya, 1979b).

Cellular death is the continuous kind of death we all pass through from birth. We all experience it all of the time. We die and are reborn, reincarnated continuously all the time. But in the West we do not think of it that way. This is the cellular death and turnover of the bone marrow, the gastrointestinal epithelium and the skin. Indeed, at the molecular level the body turns over completely every seven years. Western physiology and biochemistry are well aware of this. But the concept is not new. It is thousands of years old. However, its significance is not understood in the West. In sutra 19 we discussed host resistance and psychoneuroimmunology in terms of homeostasis, balance. To tread the spiritual path seriously (i.e. to awaken the *Kundalini*), is to shift that point of balance energetically higher and higher, to completely remodel the whole psychophysiological apparatus along with the subtle personality so that it can handle the higher flow of spiritual energies without creating imbalance leading to dysfunction or illness in the process.

Uncontrolled and involuntary death is death as we know it in the West. We know not when it will come, and when it does, it sweeps us away helplessly and beyond our control - often unconsciously. This is not a desirable good in the meditative tradition. For a master of yoga does nothing except by volition. At its core, yoga is a call for conscious living, and for conscious dying.

Controlled but involuntary death is the death of an initiate or disciple of the Tradition who has been properly prepared and who has gained some skill in the art of conscious living. The force of karma is still strong enough that the timing and manner of death remain involuntary. But once present, the disciple has varying degrees of control over the death process itself, and often enjoys the guidance of the Guru throughout to a propitious rebirth, perhaps even experiencing higher initiations and even liberation in the process. But through this control the death is peaceful and pleasant, inspiring to those present. The phrase "the pleasure and promise of death" has real practical significance here (Easwaran, 1996).

Daily meditation as death we will discuss in a moment, but *initiatory death* is an advanced form of it. This is a powerful experience of transcendence and transition, of knowing that I, the Spirit, am not this body. This is an initiatory and conscious process in yoga whereby a healthy person may experience death for a little while. Not everyone is given that experience because not everyone can withstand it. Those who are given that kind of initiation under the power of a master who can alter the state of consciousness are forever changed. Like a near death experience, the whole meaning of life for them undergoes a complete alteration.

This phenomenon is discussed in the *Kathopanishad* when the hero Nachiketas (whose name translates as the "one who does not know", ie an aspirant in the Tradition) lies at the gates of the house of the Lord of Death, Yama, (ie the Guru) for three days and three nights. When high yoga initiations take place and the master has touched his consciousness to yours, you lie at the gate of death. You do not know if you are in this body or not; you may not feel it for days, weeks or months. The consciousness is there but the body is not. You may think that you speak a whole speech, but you do not know if you are actually speaking or not, and only one word escapes your lips. You know yourself to be a being of light, looking down at this body lying there. You realize you exist, you continue, but the physical body means nothing. It is a shell. This knowledge, born of experience, takes away all fear of death, which is the principal one of the five *kleshas*, the five causes of suffering in life discussed in Patanjali's *Yogasutras* II.3 (Aranya, 1981).

Finally, there is the *death of a master which is controlled and voluntary*. A master of yoga knows the time of his death, when his mission is finished. He may announce it well ahead. When the time comes the word goes out to the close disciples, "Come! The master wants to say farewell." He takes a bath and then bathes the disciples' feet. Everyone gathers for a last meal (recall the last supper of Jesus). He may feed each disciple a morsel by hand. He then sits in the lotus posture, delivers his last lecture and final instructions. Then says farewell, draws a last breath, and drops the body consciously in a moment.

Yogic Training for Death

What kind of training must a disciple receive to be able to accomplish these feats? As embodied in Raja Yoga which is the basis of the meditative tradition, yoga is a holistic system that trains all levels of the personality at once. It trains for life as it trains for death. In other words, it trains for conscious living. The first two of the eight rungs of *ashtanga* or Raja Yoga, the *yamas* and *niyamas* - the moral do's and don'ts - are the ethical guidelines for relationships and for personal growth. They initiate right choices for the long term good (called *shreya* in the *Kathopanishad*) as opposed to the short term pleasant (called *preya* in the *Kathopanishad*), so that life has a satisfying conclusion without unresolved loose ends. It has closure. In the third limb of Raja Yoga the physical process of hatha yoga establishes the full control of consciousness and will over the psychophysical and neuromuscular systems of the body. The fourth limb, pranayama or breath control, is critical. The adept who learns to control the nasal cycle at will, to apply *sushumna* and go into the depths of meditation and remain there for hours in that state whose sign is both nostrils flowing with equal strength, such a person has no regard whatsoever for the death experience. When he has mastered *sahaja kumbhaka*, natural breath retention, he becomes aware of and controls the various energy fields in the subtle body, and in particular, the one called *udana* which controls the dying process and the final ejection of the life force from the body through the posterior fontanelle at the top of the head. The remaining internal four limbs of yoga which include meditation, are also critical, for meditation is one's daily dose of death!

Models for Death

There are two models for the death process in the perennial wisdom: sleep and meditation. Mastery of either leads to conscious control of the death process. Sleep is surprising to the Western mind; we know so little about it. The perennial wisdom, however, has a great deal to say about it.

The progressive withdrawal and interiorization of awareness as one falls asleep is considered to be a model for the same process in death. Conscious control of the process of falling asleep leads to conscious control of the same process in death. This is not our experience of sleep in the West. Sleep, surely, is not a conscious process! Indeed it can be. In the *Yogasutras* I.10 (Aranya, 1981), sleep or *nidra*, is a thought in the mind field - the thought of nothing. But the witnessing awareness can be detached from that thought so that one can fall asleep with awareness. One remains asleep producing delta waves on the EEG yet remains aware of everything in one's surroundings. Someone with this capacity does not dream and gets by with about 3 to 4 hours of sleep daily.

This is called *yoga nidra*, yogic sleep, or conscious sleep. There are a set of some 27 progressive relaxation exercises that are taught to learn it.

Relaxation exercises in yoga are carried out in the posture, *shavasana*. It is no coincidence that this word translates as the "corpse posture". When deepened, those very exercises, and progressively complex forms of them, can take one's awareness deep into the subtle body and lead to a state where it is as though the body were dead. And so the disciple is led from complexity to complexity into the experience of death and knows exactly what is going on.

The other model is meditation. The progressive withdrawal and interiorization of awareness as one goes into deep meditation is also considered to be a model for the same process in death. This is not meditation used for relaxation as is usually taught - a wonderful tool, but real meditation for the spiritual path as taught and practised by a disciple in the initiatory tradition of yoga. Meditation becomes a daily dose of death! It's ultimate aim is what is called Self-Realization - knowing that my Reality is pure Self, pure life force, pure consciousness force, that I am a Being of Light. Time and the body are transcended; neither is known and yet one is still conscious. The experience of consciousness that is aware of consciousness, of consciousness-without-an-object (Merrell-Wolffe, 1994), of pure Being that you have in meditation is your daily dose of death, your daily inoculation against death. When the hour of death comes you are so familiar with its face that it is like going into an eternal meditation. And that is both a joyful as well as a conscious and controlled process.

One who is in deep *samadhi* appears as though dead and cannot be roused. Swami Rama demonstrated these things when he was studied at the Menninger Foundation in the early 1970's. He said, "There's a secret corner in my head that I go and hide. The doctors can't find me and everyone thinks I am dead!" As a young man in India he visited a friend's house, entered the bedroom, locked the door and went into *samadhi*. When he did not appear for ten days, his concerned friends broke open the door only to find him apparently dead. When Swamiji awoke the next day he found himself in a morgue!

The mind is a field of energy which has a core or centre from which it operates and spreads out into the personality to give it life and function. At the hour of death it withdraws and returns to that centre. That centre or point then migrates like a spark to another space/time/causation set of coordinates called a re-in-carnation. Although we have not dealt with it specifically here, the philosophy of karma and reincarnation is central to all forms of the perennial wisdom. Now-a-days we call this soul recycling! To be centred in the sense meant here is another way to talk about our central theme of balance. It gets into deep topics like a personal philosophy and a life mission or purpose. The art of meditation is to learn to die in peace with centeredness. Like meditation, death is an experience of centeredness, a blessing we get at least once in life! So meditate. Learn to do it happily throughout life. And when the time for the real centeredness of death comes, you are treading familiar territory.

9. Life Planning

Whether a plan is individual or organizational, it needs to be written down in a clear way. This is for more than just effective communication or the achievement of clarity about exactly what it is one wants. For if one is unclear about what is wanted then the results will be confused and variably ineffective. The mental act of committing it to paper with clarity is part of launching the creative process itself.

Strategic planning - and life planning- is not a one time effort, but rather a cyclic and ongoing process of formulating and responding to change. The written vision becomes a dynamic document that easily adapts to and reflects this change in a timely manner. Most of the strategic planning literature deals with the world of business. Let us compare the components of a plan for an organization with individual life-planning.

The situation analysis with its internal organizational assessment combined with the macro-environmental analysis forms the basis for charting the plan of action . An organization begins by articulating a five year vision and purposes for its business. Next organizational beliefs, values, and principles that govern the way in which the vision is attained are defined. Finally, specific objectives and strategies are identified for fulfilment of the vision. This is strategic planning in very simplest terms.

The written plan will have a **mission** that states succinctly in a sentence or two exactly what business the organization is in. It is important to conceptualize this carefully. For example, are you in the business of running a railroad, or are you in the business of transportation? Although related, these are very different missions that could give rise to very different business plans. Depending on the context one may wish deliberately to conceptualize broadly (transportation) or narrowly (railroads). Sometimes the term **purpose** is used. For an organization purpose reflects its reasons for existing. It represents the value added for stakeholders as well as what makes the organization unique.

At an individual level we speak of life missions or the purpose of life and get into debates about whether they are given or discovered, or whether they are created by the individual. In this context a life mission unfolds over the person's lifetime as a co-creative venture between the ego/personality and the Centre of Consciousness. Because it unfolds over time it may seem to change as one gains life experience, as the Centre opens into awareness, and as one surrenders more and more to the guidance of the Inner Teacher. But with the wisdom that comes from the harvest of knowledge and experience in the autumn of life one can begin to view one's entire life as a unit to see the meaning and point of it all. The major events and broad themes start to emerge. One gets a sense of "the point of it all", how the grand puzzle is coming together (and the further mysteries yet to be plumbed).

It can be a useful exercise to imagine capturing the essence of the point of your life as an epitaph on your tombstone, or by imaging yourself on your death bed looking back over your life in review, or by composing a letter to your children or to your grandchildren in which you set forth the essence of your life.

A Vedic astrological chart will disclose the main influences and resources evolved from previous lives with which one began this life. Then the central mission of the life will start to come into focus, giving significance to all of its major experiences and events. One will have a sense of whether this was a life well-lived or whether one got off track, requiring a strong course correction to fulfill the final stage of the journey.

At this stage on the Path the perspective becomes transpersonal. One can think about next life planning and preparation as part of the completion of the present life. It is important to distinguish a list of personal desires along with a plan to achieve them. We understand the unfolding of a life mission as a co-creation with the Centre of Consciousness.

Beyond this broadest level of conceptualization, planning now begins to address the gap between an imagined future state born of our desires of what is wanted and a present state of where we are at now. Both individuals and organizations change with time. They unfold or evolve (or devolve). The unfolding process can have a spontaneous or organic quality to it. But this naturalness belies the careful planning and creative action that initiates it.

Many individuals confuse the idea of living in the present and being spontaneous as meaning there is no need to plan and that something out there somewhere - the Guru, the Tradition or whatever - will magically provide. This is the error of specialness referred to in sutra 57. All of us are natural creators. Act we must and therefore manifest we must. We can take control of the process and create with awareness, living and fashioning one's life like an artist. Or we can "let it happen" in which case the creating process will be unconscious and habitual with a less than satisfying result.

Yoga is skill in action, which means that the process of manifestation is carefully controlled just as a artist masters his or her medium of expression. This mastery is the true meaning of the word discipline to which so many of us are allergic.

Swami Rama worked from a cosmic vision that only a few could grasp in even a small part. Yet when it came to manifesting specific projects, both large and small, his attention to even the smallest details was amazing. Nothing was left to chance. He was a master at blending the precise requirements and action steps of manifesting with the spontaneous unfolding and synchronicity of the present moment as the universe, what he called Divine Mother, responded to his creative actions in a moment to moment dance.

This gap between the present and desired states is crossed by the construction of a vision using the faculty of imagination. A vision creates vivid images of the desired future as a depiction in pictures, symbols or words. It embodies the quality of aspiration to inspire the individual or the organization like a guiding star. What will the experience of the desired state be like in as concrete terms as possible?

Whether one works with an organizational or individual vision, the function and process are the same.

Principles are guidelines that help us translate our stated beliefs and values into decisions and behaviours. They can be expressed in sentences beginning with: "We will ...." They express the manner in which the organization does its business or the individual behaves.

We talk about whether people are "principled" in their behavours. Do they act from an ethical and moral stance or foundation in life? In contrast we talk about individuals as "unprincipled" who act selfishly and manipulate to get what they want in any way they can. In an organization such behaviour may be excused as "pragmatic" if it achieves desired results. It is further expressed in phrases like: "All's fair in love and war," or "The ends justify the means."

In the self-appraisal demanded of any spiritual aspirant one should constantly be aware of one's principles and one's underlying beliefs that govern how one acts. They need continual refinement as part of the purification of the personality. Whether for an organization or for an individual, merely stating a few high-minded principles is not enough. Stated principles should truly reflect the integrity of one's actual behaviour.

Sometimes an organization will further elaborate its underlying **beliefs and values**. Beliefs are those truths essential to supporting a vision and empowering staff.
"We belief that ..."
Values are those priorities essential to birthing and sustaining the vision.
"We value ...."

For an individual they are an elaboration of the belief systems that underlie one's principles for behaviour, and the same comments apply.

Models of the world, pictures of reality or cognitive paradigms - whatever term one uses for them - have both content and structure. Systems of values and beliefs along with cause-effects are the principal components of content. They are the source of our motivations and "make the world go around."

Some of the most profound changes that can be made in individual behaviour arise out of changing values and beliefs. They represent how the intellect makes meaning of and summarizes sensory experience. For most of us this psychic infrastructure is unconscious. We are quite unaware of what truly motivates our behaviours. We rationalize our conditioning and habitual actions with excuses, but others observe that we truly do not "walk our talk".

As discussed at the end of the core curriculum in sutra 67, accessing the Centre of Consciousness systematically can allow one to uncover the true nature of these core beliefs and values. At the level of personality these are the drivers for a life mission. Their influence can block, distort or assist co-creative activity with the Centre of Consciousness. So it is crucial to bring them into awareness and to reprogram as necessary.

Once one is clear about the business one is in, about what one desires to create in the future, and about how one plans to behave while one does it, then one is ready to work with the specifics of the plan for action. These involve goals, objectives and strategies.

Goals and objectives represent commitments to specific quantitative or observable results by a specific time that will demonstrate movement toward the vision. They are expressed as
1. A plan for ...
2. A program to ...

Goals are broader in scope and may subsume several more specific objectives as to how they might be achieved. Strategies are broad approaches and major steps to achieving goals and objectives. They address the capabilities that need to be in place to support the plan and present a succinct description of how the organization will go about achieving breakthrough results and creating a culture of continuous improvement. At the individual level goals need not be formulated in quite so elaborate a way, but the principle is the same.

New Year's resolutions are a very simple example of the basic process. In creating goals and objectives for a life mission it can be useful to address various areas of one's life such as spiritual and/or religious concerns, health and lifestyle, finances, home and family, social activities and friends, hobbies and recreation, work, travel, community service, or whatever grouping of categories makes the most sense for any given person. It is useful to write them down as well as review and revise them repeatedly.

One must restate again that this process of visioning through goal review and reformulation is what initiates the creative process. One mistake is to never write them down. Another is to write them down and never refer to them again. Then they become at best good intentions, easily forgotten as one goes off track under the demands of daily life. One day you realize that the really important things never got done and time has run out.

This raises the question of setting **priorities**. Life's possibilities are so rich that one can never do it all and one can never get it all done. The whole point of life planning is to be clear about what you really want to do, about what really matters, about what is really important in the context of a life well-lived. Here is an example of a process that can be helpful in identifying life priorities.

1. Find some paper, a pen and some uninterrupted time.
2. For five minutes only by your watch, write down all of the things you can think of that you would like to do with your life in the next five years. Brainstorm them as fast as you can write them down - all your goals and objectives. Don't stop to evaluate or critique them. Get as many down as you can in any order they come to you, no matter how trivial or wild and impossible they may seem.
   Then take one minute to group and arrange your list, adding any others that may occur to you.
3. Now repeat the process, but focus on which of these you want to accomplish in the next two years.
   Again take only a minute to revise.
4. Now imagine that your doctor has just told you that you have an incurable disease and that you have only six months to live. Take only five minutes by your watch and select out of your two year list, those items you want to accomplish in that final six months of your life.
5. Now examine the six-month list. If these are the most important things you could do with your life right now, are you working on them as your top priorities? If not, why not now?

10. Background Visioning

Twelve basic elements can be considered in constructing the larger background of one's vision (Alarius, 1991). Each one is developed in communication and co-creation with the Centre of Consciousness.

1. **Identity**. This is the end result - who you will be in this new reality you are about to manifest. Create a sovereign, magnificent identity.

2. **Relationships**. Envision a reality filled with loving relationships to the people and things in your life, to the ideas and concepts in your mind, and to your emotions.

3. **Emotional tone**. Your vision that must be filled with joy and delight, the allowing of authentic emotional expression to all beautiful things and to experiences of awe and wonder that awaken and touch the innocence within you. This authentic emotional expression is the spirit of the child within.

4. **Foundation**. Your vision will include access to all the practical resources needed to live and work in the world. It is your relationship to time, money and resources.

5. **Freedom of expression**. This quality allows you to be spontaneous in the expression of your inner Centre in a way that lets you live with excitement, intensity, adventure and drama.

6. **Making a contribution to life**. When receiving an expression of gratitude, Swami Rama would always say, "I'm just doing my duty." All contributions in your vision will come from one fundamental motivation - that your Spirit, your Centre of Consciousness, be allowed its fullest and most delighted expression. This gives rise to the metaphorical statement, "Follow your Spirit without hesitation." (Alarius, 1989).

7. **Discernment**. Your vision will include the ability to discern in each moment what is supportive to your co-creative activities, to what Spirit or the Centre of Consciousness is or is not guiding you to do from moment to moment.

8. **A sense of transpersonal power**. Once all of the above things are in place, you will have a consistent experience of background transpersonal power, of the power of your Centre of Consciousness.

9. **A consistent experience of wholeness**. You will have an allowing and unconditional loving relationship to all that you are, the good and the bad, the ugly and beautiful, the petty and magnificent. Only in this way can you allow yourself the experience of your wholeness.

10. **Access to other dimensions**. Your vision will allow you to have constant and easy access to higher truth through the Centre of Consciousness.

11 **Congruence of systems.** In your vision all the systems that spontaneously emerge in your life (religious, spiritual, economic and cultural), will arise in your own consciousness from the Centre of Consciousness. Only in this way can you function with mastery of divine manifestation and expression in a world of form.

12. **Service to the tradition.** In your vision you will be completely and transpersonally dedicated to the fulfillment of the higher mission of the Tradition of the Himalayan Masters (what is called Guru's mission in yoga) or whatever other spiritual lineage you may express. This is one of the implications of initiation and acceptance as a disciple within a lineage or tradition of spiritual expression. Every disciple has his or her unique, individualistic expression of that mission, but each will be dedicated to that group intention. The Bodhisattwa vow is an example.

From these components one can begin to see the grandeur and breadth of a transpersonal vision. The background vision not only sets the context and foundation for the foreground - the background stage set for the actor who plays the role in the foreground, but also is the enabler of the life mission and a profound attractor for the necessary synchronicities that will guide its manifestation.

Glossary

abhyasa	Regular practice.
adhikara	Qualification.
advaita	Non-dualism; in vedanta, the unity of the Self (Atman) with Brahman.
ahamkara	Ego.
ahimsa	Nonviolence.
anamayakosha	Physical (food) sheath or body.
ananda	Bliss.
anandamayakosha	Blissful sheath or body.
anantarya	Transition in a sequence.
antar mouna	The practice of inner silence.
apara vidya	Lower intellectual knowledge of the manifested world.
aparigraha	Non-possessiveness.
ashtanga	Eight-fold.
asteya	Non-stealing.
astik	Belief in Truth.
atha	Now.
atman	The inner divine Self.
atma shakti	Spiritual energy, force.
avidya	Ignorance.
ayurveda	Ancient Indian medical science.
bhakti yoga	The yoga of devotion.
bhava	Attitude.
bindu	Drop, point
brahmacharya	Continence, celibacy.
brahman	The ultimate Reality. God the Father. Logos, the transcendental reality.
brahma-vihara	Frolicking in God.
buddhi	Intelligence, understanding.
cidakasha	Inner or mental space.
cit	Consciousness.
chakra, cakra	Wheel, plexus, centre.
chandra, candra	Moon.
chayapurusha	Shadow man; an advanced form of meditation on one's shadow.
chitta, citta	Mind, memory.
chitta shakti	Mental energy.
daksha	Intelligence.
dama	Restraint of the senses.
darshan	Audience with a holy individual.
dharana	Concentration.
dharma	Law, duty.
dhyana	Meditation.
dvesha	Aversion.
grahitr	Knower.
grahya	Object to be known.

grahana	Instrument of knowing.
guna	Quality, attribute, characteristic, constituent of prakrti or primal nature composed of (depending on individual school's interpretations) the three aspects: sattva, which is buoyant, light, illuminating, knowledge, and happiness; rajas, which is stimulating, mobile, pain, and action; and tamas, which is heavy, enveloping, indifferent, and laziness.
Hiranyagarbha	Golden womb. God, the immanent spirit of the universe.
hitam	Beneficial.
ida	Subtle nadi running parallel to the spinal column. It controls the breath in the left nostril, and when dominant one's behaviour is intuitive and passive.
irshya	Jealousy.
Ishvara	The Lord. The personal God.
Ishvara pranidhana	Surrender to God.
jitendriya	Control over the senses.
jiva	Individual soul.
jnana yoga	Yoga of Knowledge.
kama	Passion.
karanasharira	Causal body.
karma	Action that leads to results through the law of cause and effect.
karma yoga	Yoga of action.
karuna	Compassion.
klesha	Affliction.
kosha	Sheath, body.
kriya	Action, activity; kriya yoga is a path of action.
krodha	Anger.
kundalini	"The serpent power"; spiritual or evolutionary energy.
lila	The divine game of God who creates the worlds in play.
lobha	Greed.
mada	Pride, frenzy.
maitri	Friendship.
mahasamadhi	Death of a Yoga Master.
manana	Reflection, consideration
manas	Lower mind that registers and stores sensory impressions.
manomayakosha	Mental sheath or body.
mantram	A holy phrase or spiritual formula; combination of syllables or words corresponding to a particular energy vibration and used as an object for meditation.
matsarya	Malice, small-mindedness.
maya	Worldly illusion.
mitam	Measured.
moha	Delusion, attachment.
mudita	Happiness.
nadi	Subtle energy channel.

neti neti	Not this, not that.
nididhyasana	Meditation; contemplation. Continuous, unbroken stream of ideas of the same kind as those of Brahman.
nidra	Sleep.
niyamas	Observances.
pada	Chapter.
para vidya	Higher or transcendental knowledge.
parikarma	Purification.
pingala	Subtle nadi running parallel to the spinal column. It controls the flow of the breath in the right nostril, and when dominant, one's behaviour is rational, active and energetic.
prajna	Wisdom of the Self. Wisdom. Intuitive wisdom.
prakriti	Nature.
pramana	True conceptual knowledge.
prana	Subtle vital energy.
pranamayakosha	Subtle energy sheath or body.
prana shakti	Vital life force.
prana vidya	Science of prana.
pranayama	Breath control; Voluntary control or expansion of the pranic force.
pratyahara	Withdrawal of the senses.
preya	The pleasant.
priyam	Pleasant.
purashcharana	Special intensive practice of a mantra for self-purification and liberation, to attain a desired result, or to attain the siddhis of that mantra - usually the number of syllables multiplied by a hundred thousand plus twenty percent.
purusha	Spirit, individual soul, roughly interchangeable with the Atman.
raga	Attachment.
raja yoga	The Royal Path as taught by Patanjali in his Yogasutras.
rajas	See guna.
rasayanas	Ayurvedic rejuvenation practices.
saccidananda	Existence, consciousness and bliss.
sadhaka	Spiritual aspirant.
sadhana	Spiritual practice.
sahaja	Natural, spontaneous state of spiritual awareness.
sahasrara	Thousand petaled lotus; seventh chakra at the crown of the head.
sakshatkara	Self-realization; direct experience.
sakshi caitanya	Cit; absolute, unbounded or universal consciousness.
samadhana	Freedom from conflicts.
samadhi	Absorption.
samahitam	No question remains unanswered.
sambhogakaya	One of the three sheaths of the Buddha; the subtle sheath of enjoyment in which a Buddha or Bodhisattva dwells on the earth or beyond. The enlightened universal spirit immanent in the universe.
samsara	Earthly existence.
samskaras	Subtle unconscious residues; personality traits conditioned over one or many lives.
samyama	Dharana, dhyana and samadhi used together.
santosha	Contentment.

sarva hinsa vinirmukta	Abstention from violence.
sahaja	Spontaneous, natural.
sahaja kumbhaka	Natural breath retention.
sahasrara	Thousand petalled lotus.
sakshi caitanya	Cit. Witness. Absolute or pure universal consciousness.
sat	Existence.
sat cit ananda	Existence, consciousness and bliss.
sattva	See guna.
satya	Truth.
satyagraha	Gandhi's term for non-violent, moral struggle.
shakti	Power, force.
shaktipat	Higher spiritual initiation.
shama	Quietude.
shantih	Peace.
shatsampat	Six treasures.
shaucha	Purity.
shavasana	Corpse posture for relaxation.
Shiva	A major deity of the Hindu Pantheon and the third god of the Hindu Trinity. Consciousness as the male and passive aspect of God as opposed to Shakti as power and the feminine, active and manifesting aspect of God.
shraddha	Faith.
shravana	Hearing a discourse; study.
shreya	The good.
shuchi	Purity.
siddhi	Accomplishment, perfection, achievement; advanced powers that unfold during the practice of yoga.
sthula-sharira	Physical body.
suksma-sharira	Subtle body.
sumeru	mountain; referring to the spine.
surya	Sun.
sushumna	The central nadi running along the spinal column from its base to the crown of the head. When dominant both nostrils flow equally and the mind becomes quiet and pleasant and can attain deep meditation.
sutratma	The "thread-soul"; in vedanta the soul that passes like a thread through the universe.
svadhyaya	Self-study.
svara yoga	The science of the breath and the subtle energies.
svarupa	Essential nature.
tamas	See guna.
tapas	Austerity.
titiksha	Forbearance.
turiya	The fourth state of consciousness; supreme consciousness, absolute reality.
udana	One of the five pranas on the subtle body.
uparati	Withdrawal from worldly interests.
upeksha	Indifference towards the evil in others.
vairagya	Detachment, non-attachment.

vanaprastha	The third ashrama or period of life corresponding to early retirement.
veda	Body of knowledge; the most ancient revealed Sanskrit scriptures.
vidya	Science or branch of study; knowledge, wsidom.
vijnanamayakosha	Buddhi; intellectual or intuitive sheath or body.
vritti caitanya	Citta; phenomenal, modified or bound consciousness.
yamas	Restraints.
yoga	Union with God; a path or discipline leading to complete integration of consciousness or Self-realization.
yoga nidra	Yogic sleep.
yogasutras	Manual on raja yoga written by the sage, Patanjali, around 200 B.C.

Bibliography

Alarius (1988) The Force of Wisdom: Three Radical Shifts into Divine Expression. Earth Mission Publishing, Sedona AZ (audiotapes).

Alarius (1989) Following Spirit: Transcending the Illusion of Resistance. Earth Mission Publishing, Sedona AZ (audiotapes).

Alarius and Polaria (1990) Emergence: The Co-Creation of Heaven on Earth.. Earth Mission Publishing, Sedona AZ (audiotapes).

Alarius (1991) Genesis: The Solar Vision Technique. Earth Mission Publishing, Sedona AZ (audiotapes).

Alpert R/Ram Dass (1982) A ten year perspective. Journal of Transpersonal Psychology 14:171-183.

Andreas S, Andreas C (1987) Change Your Mind and Keep the Change. Advanced Submodalities Interventions. Real People Press, Moab, Utah.

Aranya, Swami Hariharananda (1981) Yoga Philosophy of Patanjali, University of Calcutta, Calcutta, India.

Arya, Pandit Usharbudh (1979a) God. Himalayan Institute Press, Honesdale PA.

Arya Pandit Usharbudh (1979b) Meditation and the Art of Dying. Himalayan Institute Press, Honesdale PA.

Arya, Pandit Usharbudh (1981) Mantra and Meditation. Himalayan Institute Press, Honesdale PA.

Arya, Pandit Usharbudh (1986) Yoga-Sutras of Patanjali, Vol. 1. Himalayan Institute Press, Honesdale PA.

Aurobindo Ghose, Sri (1972) On Himself. All India Press, Pondicherry, India.

Aurobindo Ghose, Sri (1971) Letters on Yoga (Vols. 1-3). All India Press, Pondicherry, India.

Ballentine, RM (1999) Radical Healing. Integrating the World's Great Therapeutic Traditions to Create a New Transformative Medicine. Harmony Books, New York.

Bandler R (1985) Using Your Brain - for a Change. Real People Press, Moab, Utah.

Bandler R, Grinder J (1982) Reframing. Real People Press, Moab, Utah.

Becker RO, Selden G (1985) The Body Electric: Electromagnetism and the Foundation of Life. William Morrow & Co., New York.

Benson H, Beary JF, Carol MP (1974) The relaxation response. Psychiatry 37:37.

Bhagavad Gita. Translation by Swami Rama (1985) Perennial Philosophy of the Bhagavad Gita. Himalayan Institute Press, Honesdale PA.

Bohm D (1983) Wholeness and the Implicate Order. Routledge, Chapman & Hall, New York.

Bohm D, Peat DF (1987) Science, Order, and Creativity. Bantam, New York.

Brennan BA (1987) Hands of Light. A Guide to Healing Through the Human Energy Field. Bantam Books, New York.

Brennan BA (1993) Light Emerging. The Journey of Personal Healing. Bantam Books, New York.

Brunton P. (1988) The Notebooks of Paul Brunton (Vol. 15), Advanced Contemplation/The Peace Within You. Larson Publications, Burdett, New York.

Bruyere R (1989) Wheels of Light: A Study of the Chakras. Bon Publications, Arcadia CA.

Cameron-Bandler (1985) Solutions. FuturePace Inc. San Rafael, CA.

Capra F (1991) The Tao of Physics. Ed. 3. Shambala, Boston.

Capra F (1996) The Web of Life. A New Scientific Understanding of Living Systems. Anchor Books, Doubleday, New York.

Carroll L (1998) Kryon Book Six: Partnering With God. The Kryon Writings, Inc., Del Mar CA

Chalmers AF (1982) What is This Thing Called Science. University of Queensland Press, St. Lucia, Queensland, Australia.

Childre D & Martin H (1999) The HeartMath Solution. HarperCollins, New York.

Churchland PS (1986) Neurophilosophy. Toward a Unified Science of the Mind-Brain. The MIT Press, Cambridge, Massachusetts.

Clegg SR, Hardy C, Nord WR (Eds) (1996) Handbook of Organization Studies. Sage Publications, Thousand Oaks CA.

Collins M (1976) Light on the Path; Through the Gates of Gold. Theosophical University Press, Pasadena CA.

Combs A. (1995) The Radiance of Being. Complexity, Chaos and the Evolution of Consciousness. Paragon House, St. Paul, Minnesota.

Course in Miracles (1975) Foundation for Inner Peace, Tiburon CA.

Damasio A (1999) The Feeling of What Happens. Body and Emotion in the Making of Consciousness. Harcourt and Brace, New York.

Dilts R, Grinder J, Bandler R, Bandler LC, Delozier J (1979) Neuro-Linguistic Programming I, Meta Pubs, Cupertino CA.

Easwaren, Eknath (1975) The End of Sorrow. The Bhagavad Gita for Daily Living, Volume I. Nilgiri press, Petaluma CA.

Easwaren, Eknath (1978) Meditation. An Eight-Point Program. Nilgiri press, Petaluma CA.

Easwaran, Eknath (1992) Dialogues with Death. A Journey Through Consciousness. Nilgiri Press, Tomales CA.

Easwaran, Eknath (1996) The Undiscovered Country. Exploring the Promise of Death. Nilgiri Press, Tomales CA.

Evans-Wentz WY (1960) The Tibetan Book of the Dead. Oxford Univ Press, London.

Faivre A & Needleman J (Eds) (1992) Modern Esoteric Spirituality. Crossroad, New York.

Freedman J, Combs G. Narrative Therapy (1996) The Social Construction of Preferred Realities. WW Norton & Co, New York.

Freemantle F & Chögyam Trungpa (1975) The Tibetan Book of the Dead. The Great Liberation Through Hearing in the Bardo. Shambhala, Boulder CO.

Gallo F (1999) Energy Psychology: Explorations at the Interface of Energy, Cognition, Behavior and Health. CRC Press, Boca Raton FL.

Ghiselin B (1985) The Creative Process: A Symposium. New American Library, New York.

Goodwin JS and Goodwin JM (1984) The Tomato Effect: Rejection of highly efficacious therapies. J Am Med Assoc 11:2387-2390.

Gopi Krishna (1971) Kundalini: The Evolutionary Energy in Man. Shambhala, Boulder CO.

Gopi Krishna (1974) Higher Consciousness and Kundalini. F.I.N.D. Research Trust, Ontario.

Goswami A (1995) The Self-Aware Universe. How Consciousness Creates the Material World. GP Putnam's Sons, New York.

Grinder J, Bandler R (1975) Structure of Magic. Vol I. Science and Behaviour Books, Palo Alto CA.

Grinder J, Bandler R (1976) Structure of Magic. Vol II. Science and Behaviour Books, Palo Alto CA.

Grof C, Grof S (1989) Spiritual Emergency: When Personal Transformation Becomes a Crisis. Jeremy P Tarcher, Los Angeles.

Grof C, Grof S (1990) The Stormy Search for the Self: A Guide to Personal Growth Through Transformational Crisis. Jeremy P Tarcher, Los Angeles.

Guyton AC and Hall JE (Eds) (1996) Textbook of Medical Physiology. 9th Ed. WB Saunders Co, Philadelphia. P742.

Harman W (1988) Global Mind Change. Knowledge Systems, Inc., Indianapolis IN.

Henatsch H-D (1996) Appendix. Psychomotor Aspects of the Brain-MindProblem. Pp1091-93 in Greger R and Windhorst U (Eds) (1996) Comprehensive Human Physiology. From Cellular Mechanisms to Integration. Springer-Verlag, Heidelberg.

Hicks J, Hicks E (1988, 1991) A New Beginning I and II. Abraham-Hicks Publishers, San Antonio TX.

Huxley A (1944) The Perennial Philosophy. Harper and Row, New York.

Indich WM (1995) Consciousness in Advaita Vedanta. Motilal Banarsidass, Delhi.

James T, Woodsmall W (1988) Time Line Therapy and the Basis of Personality. Meta Publications, Cupertino CA.

James W (1890) The Principles of Psychology, Vols 1 & 2. Reprinted by Dover Publications, New York.

James W (1902/1929) The Varieties of Religious Experience. Modern Library, New York.

Jerry LM (1985) Paradigm Shifts in Clinical Research: The Tomato Effect

Revisited. Clinical and Investigative Medicine 8:249-250.

Jerry M (1996) Psychoneuroimmunology. Chapter 87 in R Greger & U Windhorst (eds) Comprehensive Human Physiology, Vol 2. Springer-Verlag, Berlin.

Johari, Harish (1986) Tools for Tantra. Destiny Books, Vermont.

Johnston VS (1999) Why We Feel. The Science of Human Emotions. Perseus Books, Reading MA.

Kafatos M & Nadeau R (1990) The Conscious Universe. Part and Whole in Modern Physical Theory. Springer-Verlag, New York.

Kathopanishad. Translation by Swami Nikhilananda (1977) The Upanishads, Vol 1. Ramakrishna-Vivekananda Center, New York.

Khan, Pir Vilayat Inayat (1999) Awakening. A Sufi Experience. Jeremy P Tarcher, New York.

Koertge N (1998) A House Built on Sand. Exposing Postmodern Myths about Science. Oxford, University Press, Oxford, England.

Korzybski A (1980) Science and Sanity. An Introduction to Non-Aristotelian Systems and General Semantics. Ed 4. The International Non-Aristotelian Library Pub. Co.

Kristof A, Emami H (1999) Enlightenment Beyond Traditions. The Complete Inner Map of Spiritual Awakening. Motilal Banarsidass Publishers, Delhi.

Kuhn TS (1962) The Structure of Scientific Revolutions. Ed 2. University of Chicago Press, Chicago.

Lax WD (1996) Narrative, Social Constructionism, and Buddhism. Pp195-220 in Rosen H & Kuehlwein KT (Eds) (1996). Constructing Realities. Meaning-Making Perspectives for Psychotherapists. Jossey-Bass Publishers, San Francisco.

Lovejoy A (1936) The Great Chain of Being. Harvard University Press, Cambridge, Mass.

MacLean PD (1984) Psychosomatic Disease and the Visceral Brain. Recent Developments Bearing on the Papez Theory of Emotions. In Basic Readings in Neurophysiology, RL Isaacson (Ed.) Harper and Row, Inc., New York, pp181-211.

Maturana H & Varela F (1980) Autopoiesis and Cognition. D Reidel, Dordrecht, Holland.

Maturana H & Varela F (1998) Ed 2. The Tree of Knowledge. The Biological Roots of Human Understanding. Shambala, Boston.

Merrell-Wolff F (1994) Experience and Philosophy. A personal record of transformation and a discussion of transcendental consciousness. State University of New York Press, Albany.

MSI (1996) Ascension. An Analysis of the Art of Ascension as Taught by the Ishayas. Society for Ascension, Waynesville NC.

Nelson J (1994) Healing the Spirit: A New Understanding of the Crisis and Treatment of the Mentally Ill. Jeremy P Tarcher, Los Angeles.

Niranjanananda, Paramahansa (1992) Prashnopanishad. Deoghar, Bihar, India.

Nuernberger P (1979) Freedom from Stress. Himalayan Institute Press, Honesdale PA

O'Connor J and Seymour J (1990) Introductory Neuro-Linguistic Programming. Aquarian Press, Cornwall, England.

Papez JW (1937) A Proposed Mechanism of Emotion. Arch. Neurol. Psychiat. 38:725-743.

Paramahansa Yogananda (1983) Autobiography of a Yogi. Self-Realization Fellowship, Los Angeles, CA.

Pert CB (1997) Molecules of Emotion. Why You Feel the Way You Feel. Scribner, New York.

Pierrakos JC (1975) The Energy Field in Man and Nature. Institute for the New Age, New York.

Prakash P (1998) The Yoga of Spiritual Devotion. A Modern Translation of the Narada Bhakti Sutras. Inner Traditions International, Rochester, VT.

Pribram K (1991) Brain and Perception: Holonomy and Structure in Figural Processing. Erlbaum, Hillsdale N.J.

Purves D et al (1997) Neuroscience. Sinauer Associates, Sunderland MA.

Redfield J (1993) The Celestine Prophesy. Warner Books, New York, New York.

Rosen H & Kuehlwein KT (Eds) (1996). Constructing Realities. Meaning-Making Perspectives for Psychotherapists. Jossey-Bass Publishers, San Francisco.

Rossi EL (1986) Altered states of consciousness in everyday life: The ultradian rhythms. pp97 in: Wolman BB and Ullman M (Eds) Handbook of States of Consciousness. Van Nostrand Reinhold Co., New York

Rossi EL (1993) The Psychobiology of Mind-Body Healing. New Concepts of Therapeutic Hypnosis. Revised Ed. Norton & Co, New York

Rossi EL, Cheek BD (1988) Mind-Body Therapy. Methods of Ideodynamic Healing in Hypnosis. WW Norton & Co., New York.

Scott WR (1995) Institutions and Organizations. Theory and Research. Sage Publications, Thousand Oaks CA.

Selye H (1976) The Stress of Life. McGraw-Hill, New York.

Slife BD, Williams RN (1995) What's Behind the Research? Discovering Hidden Assumptions in the Behavioral Sciences. Sage Publications, Thousand Oaks CA.

Smith H (1982) Beyond the Post-Modern Mind. Theosophical Pub., Wheaton, Illinois.

Sokal A & Bricmond J (1998) Fashionable Nonsense. Postmodern Philosophers' Abuse of Science. St. Martins Press.

Sperry R and Gazzaniga M (1967) Language following disconnection of the hemispheres. pp 177 in: C Millikan and F Darley (Eds). Brain mechanisms underlying speech and language. Grune and Stratton, New York.

Stapp, HP (1993) Mind, Matter, and Quantum Mechanics. Springer-Verlag, Berlin.

Swami Muktibodhananda Saraswati (1983) Swara Yoga. The Tantric Science of Brain Breathing. Bihar School of Yoga, Munger, Bihar, India.

Swami Muktibodhananda Saraswati (1985) Hatha Yoga Pradipika. The Light on Hatha Yoga. Bihar School of Yoga, Munger, Bihar, India.

Swami Nikhilananda (1977a) Ed. 4 The Upanishads. A New Translation. 4 Volumes. Ramakrishna-Vivekananda Center, New York.

Swami Nikhilananda (1977b) Ed. 4 The Upanishads. A New Translation. Volume 1. Ramakrishna-Vivekananda Center, New York.

Swami Nikhilananda (1987) Ed 5 The Mandukya Upanishad. Advaita Ashrama, Calcutta.

Swami Niranjanananda Saraswati (1994) Prana, Pranayama, Prana Vidya. Bihar School of Yoga, Munger, Bihar, India.

Swami Rama (1976) Life Here and Hereafter. Himalayan Institute Press, Honesdale PA.

Swami Rama, Ballentine R, Ajaya S (1976a) Yoga and Psychotherapy. The Evolution of Consciousness. Himalayan Institute Press, Honesdale PA.

Swami Rama (1982a) Enlightenment Without God. Mandukya Upanishad. Himalayan Institute Press, Honesdale PA.

Swami Rama (1982b) Choosing a Path. Himalayan Institute Press, Honesdale PA.

Swami Rama (1985) Perennial Philosophy of the Bhagavad Gita. Himalayan Institute Press, Honesdale PA.

Swami Rama (1986a) Path of Fire and Light I. Advanced Practices of Yoga. Himalayan International Institute, Honesdale, PA.

Swami Rama (1986b) Love Whispers. Himalayan International Institute, Honesdale, PA.

Swami Rama (1992) Meditation and Its Practice. Himalayan International Institute, Honesdale, PA.

Swami Rama (1996) Sacred Journey. Living Purposefully and Dying Gracefully. Himalayan International Institute of Yoga Science and Philosophy, New Delhi, India.

Swami Rama (1999a). Mastery Over Death. Himalayan Institute Hospital Trust Bulletin VII(I):1-3, June.

Swami Rama (1999b). Guru Purnima Talk Reprinted by the Himalayan Institute Hospital Trust, Jolly Grant, Dehradun, India.

Swami Satyananda Saraswati (1975) Meditations from the Tantras. Bihar School of Yoga, Munger, Bihar, India.

Swami Satyananda Saraswati (1989) Four Chapters on Freedom: Commentary on Yoga Sutras of Patanjali. Bihar School of Yoga, Munger, Bihar, India.

Swami Veda Bharati (1998) The Himalayan Tradition of Yoga Meditation. Sadhana Mandir Trust, Rishikesh, India.

Swami Vishnu Devananda (1978) Meditation and Mantras. OM Lotus Publishing Company, New York, New NY.
Talbot M (1981) Mysticism and the New Physics. Bantam, New York.
The Mother (1972) Questions and Answers: 1950-1951. Sri Aurobindo Ashram Press, Pondicherry, India.
The Mother (1979) Health and Healing in Yoga. Selections from the writings and talks of the Mother. Sri Aurobindo Ashram, Pondicherry, India.
Thie J (1996) Touch for Health. DeVorss Publications, Marina del Ray CA.
Tigunait, Pandit Rajmani (1993) The Tradition of the Himalayan Masters. Himalayan Institute Press. Honesdale PA.
Tigunait Pandit Rajmani (1996) The Power of Mantra and the Mystery of Initiation. Yoga International Books, Honesdale PA.
Tigunait, Pandit Rajmani (1998) Swami Rama of the Himalayas. His life and Mission. Himalayan Institute Press, Honesdale,
Tipler FJ (1994) The Physics of Immortality. Modern Cosmology, God and the Resurrection of the Dead. Doubleday, New York.
Tsongkapa (1995). Preparing for Tantra: The Mountain of Blessings. Paljor Publications, Delhi.
Tripura Rahasya. Translation by Swami Sri Ramanananda Saraswathi (1980). TN Venkataraman Pub., Tiruvannamalai, India.
Varela F & Coutinho A (1991) Second Generation Immune Networks. Immunology Today **12**:159-166.
Varela F, Thompson E & Rosch E (1991) The Embodied Mind. MIT Press, Cambridge, Mass.
Werntz D, Bickford R, Bloom F, Singh-Khalsa S (1982) Alternating Cerebral Hemispheric Activity and Lateralization of Autonomic Nervous Function. Neurobiology $\underline{4}$: 225.
Walsh (1979) Meditation Research: An introduction and review. Journal of Transpersonal Psychology 11:161-174.
Washburn M (1995) The Ego and the Dynamic Ground. A Transpersonal Theory of Human Development. Ed.2 SUNY, Albany
Wilber K (1983) Eye to Eye. Doubleday/Anchor, New York.
Wilber K (1987) Ken Wilber: An interview by Catherine Ingram. Yoga Journal 76:38-49, (September/October).
Wilber K (1996) A Brief History of Everything. Shambala, Boston.
Yoga Vasishtha. Translation by Swami Venkatesananda (1993) Vasistha's Yoga. State University of New York Press, Albany.
Yogananda P (1995) The Bhagavad Gita. Self-Realization Fellowship, Los Angeles CA.
Zukov G (1979) The Dancing Wu Li Masters: An Overview of the New Physics. Bantam, New York.

Index

Where possible entries are indexed under sutras for appreciation of the full context of the concept.
p100 means page 100; s71 means sutra 71; n6 means end note 6.

abhyasa, p22, s49, s65, s68
absorption, s65, s90
action, s60, s79, s96
acupuncture, s18
ahamkara, s21
alignment, s86, s87
ananda, s23
aparavidya, s24
apotheosis, s58
appreciation, s48
"as if," s64, s82, s85
ascension, p16, p18, s93
At-one-ment, s89
Atman, see Self
Atma shakti, s20
attachment, s50
Attunement, s68 - s99
aura, s18
autonomic nervous system (ANS), s17, s19, s20, s21
ayurveda, s6

background visioning, s83, s86, n10
beliefs, s22, s61, s62, s63, s67, s76, s77, s82, s83, s84, s85
Bhagavad Gita, s5, s36, s66
Bhakti Yoga, p23, s65, s74, s92
Bharati lineage, p21
bhava, s65
blame, s64
blessings, s100 - s108
bliss, s50, s53, s65
body (physical), s15 - s17
brahmacharya, s10
brahma-viharas, s13, s59
breath, s19, s20, s23
buddhi, s21, s61, s62, s63, s68
butterfly effect, s59

Centre of Consciousness, p15, s24, s29, s30, s31, s34 - s40, s41, s53, s61 - s63, s65, s67, s69 - s71, s76, s78, s81 - s83, s85 - s89, s91, s95 - s100, s105, s107
  ascension, and, p18, s93
  sat cit ananda, as, s15, s16, s24, s48
  awakening, and, s29
  channelling of, p19, s56, s67
  consciousness-with-an-object, and s24
  consciousness-without-an-object, as, s24, s26, s35, s37
  definition of, s1
  direct knowing of, s34, s35
  disturbance with awakening, and, p18, s88
  God, relationships to, s38, s39, s40, s41
  guru, and, s39
  inner ashram, and, s12, s41
  inner teacher, and, s38, s39
  intuition, and, s20, s38
  love, and, s38
  meditation, and, p26
  mystical experience of, s28-s38
  non-recognition of, s30, s31
  Now, and, s35, s39
  personality, and, s15, s16
  plenum, as, s36
  Presence, as, s36, s37, s39
  samahita yoga, and, p15
  Silence, as, s37, s40
  Space, as, s37
  Void, as, s37
  Warrior Within, as, s40
  worship of, s107

cerebral dominance, s19, s20
chakras, s15, s16, s18, s20
chandra svara, s20
channelling, s56, s67
chain of being, s14
chariot of *sadhana*, s65, s68, s93
chitta, s21, s23
chitta shakti, s20
choosing a path, s94
co-creative partnering, s83
cognition, s21, s22, s76
coherence, s48, n3
commitment, s12, s13, s45, s47, s51, s87, s101
common sense, s62

communication, s38
communion, s89
compelling reference experience, s22
concentration, s26, s28, s38, s84, s87, s89, s90, s102 - 108
consciousness, s15, s16, s18, s23, s24, s26
   Advaita Vedanta, in, n6
   scientific study of, n6
consciousness-with-an-object, s24, s90, n6
consciousness-without-an-object, s24, s 35, s37, s90, n6
contemplation, s20
curriculum, s48 - s67, p93, p132
cybernetics, s22

death, p30, s47, s58, n8
deletion, linguistic, s21, s22
dependency, s60
desire, s60, s65, s87
desirelessness, s65
detachment, see nonattachment
devotion, s68 - s75
dharana, see concentration
diaphragmatic breathing, s20
disciples, s12
discipleship, s42, s45
discipline, s68, s88, s101
discrimination, s62, s94, s103
distortion, linguistic, s21, s22
disturbance (with awakening), s31
dvesha, s21, s22
duty, s60

ego, s22, p27, s49, s51, s61 - s63, s82
emergent properties, s2
emotions, s21, s22, s55, s85
   neurophysiology of, s5, s6, n1
   purification of, s10, s22, p24
   tone of, s59
enlightenment, s8, p16, p17, s81, s82
   false, s44
energy, s15, s16, s53, s55, s59
   fields, s18, s26
   medicine, s18, s26
   psychology, s25, s88
equanimity, s104
evolutionary synergies, s50
external behaviour, s21

faith, s49, s56, s85
feedback, s64, s76

feelings, s55, n1
field coupling, s18
figures, fig 1 - s10, s11, p45
     fig 2 - s15, s16, p54
     fig 3 - s21, p63
     fig 4 - s92, p169
foreground visioning, s86, n10
freedom, s51

generalization, linguistic, s21
generosity, s50
genius, s52
Golden Womb, see *Hiranyagarbha*
grace, s69, s70, s71, s101, s108
gratitude, s48
guidance, s87
guilt, s64
guru, p15, s53 - s55, s58, s69, s70 - s72, s74, s75, s100, s108
guru-disciple relationship, s39, s40 - s43, s45, s66, s100

happiness, s48
healing, s52
health, s67
high sensory perception, s18
Himalayan Tradition, s4, p21, s61, s93, s95
Hiranyagarbha, p15, s72, s75
holographic universe, s23, s67, n4
holomovement, s23
Holy Ghost, p16
homeostasis, s5, s6, s19, s22
humility, s57, s82
hypnosis, s19

ida, s18, s20
identity, s79, s82
identity shift, s47, s51, s61 - s63, s81, s82, s89 - s91
illness, s18, s20, s21
imagery, s21, s22
imagination, s80
immune system, s17
inertia, s85
initiation, s3, p21, s27, s53, s69 - s71, s75, s93, s95, s99, s100
inner sounds, s65
Inner Teacher, s2, p15, p21, p23, s47, s55, s66, s72, s99, s100
intuitive diagnosis, s18
integration, s53
integrity, s49, s103

intentionality, s85, s87, s97
internal computation, s21
internal behaviour, s21
internal states, s21
intuition, p19, p20, s39, s52, s54 - s56, s67, s98
involution, s2
Ishvara, s72, s73, s74
Ishvara pranadhana, s11 - s13, p22, s49, s65, s72, s75

jiva, s68
Jnana Yoga, s11, s15, s17, p23, p27, s54, s67, s92
joy, s48
judgement, s51

karma, p17, s24, s58, s59, s76, s83, s87
Karma Yoga, s12, p16, s21, p23, s48 - s50, s60, s76 -s87, s92
kinesiology, p24, s67
koshas, see sheaths
kriya yoga, s11, s12
kundalini, s6, p19

language, s21, s22, s54
law of attraction, s59, s79, s83
learning, s64
life planning, n9
    background visioning, and, n10
life transitions, s1
Light, see Centre of Consciousness
light, inner, s52
limitation, s82, s84
limbic system, s6, n1
love, s48, s50, s96
    unconditional, s50, s51
lunar cycles, s20

macrocosm, s24
manana, p28
manas, s21
manifestation, s59, s60, s75, s76, s80, s81, s84 - s87
    background, s79, n10
    foreground, s79
mantra, s12, p25, p26, s93, s95
matter (physical), s23, s24
maya, s22, s23, s32
meditation s21, p25, p26, s27, s53, s65, s88 - s99, s107
    in action s65, s89, s98
    on the Centre of Consciousness s99, p178
    side effects of, s88

meridian therapies, p24, s88
metaphysics, s23, s27
microcosm, s24
millennium, p16
mind, s21 - s23, s39, s68, s104
    contents of, s55
    energy field, as, s54
mission, life, s51, s79
models of the world, s9, s12, s17, s21, s22, p24, p26, s51, s55, s59, s76, s77, s82 - s85
    beliefs, and, s17
    five senses, and, s17
models, utility of, s21
morality, s7, s9
mystical experience, s28 - s47
    Centre of Consciousness, of, s28 - s38

Nada Yoga, s65
nadis, s18, s20
nadi shodhanam, s20
near death experience, s58
negativity, s59
narrative, s22
neurocardiology, s17, p23, n3
nididhyasana, p29
niyamas, s9, p26, figure 1
nonattachment, s10, p23, s46, s49, s65, s69, s70, s71, s77, s79, s83, s97, s105
nostril dominance, s19, s20
non-violence, s10
Now, s54

objective experience, s28
OM, s72
opportunity, s100, s101

paradigms, s22, s27, s76, s84
    life planning, and, s78, n9, n10
    paradigm blindness, s27
    paradigm shifts, s27, s77
    see also models of the world
parikarmas, s59
parasympathetic nervous system (PNS), s17
paravidya, s24
path, the short, s82
perception, s21
perennial wisdom, s14, p17
personal boundaries, s61 - s63
personality, s14, s24, s27
    divinization of, s53
    subpersonalities, s49

Vedantic model, s15, s16, figure 2
philosophy of life, p27
physical body, s18
physics, s15, s16
pingala, s18, s20
planetary transition, p16, p18, s93
planning, life, n9
    background visioning, and, n10
positivity, s59
possum response, s17
postmodernism, s22, s26
practice, s65
practising the presence of God, s65, s99
prana, s18, s26
prana shakti, s20
pranayama, s18
prana vidya, s18
pratyahara, p25
prerequisites, s6, s7
Presence, s51, s65, s66, s97
pride, s57
projection, s84
protection, s61
psychics, s55
psychoneuroimmunology (PNI), s17, s21, s22, p23, s77, n2
psychosomatic network, s24
psychosomatic illness, s18
purification, s6, s22, s69, s70, s71, s88, s105
Purusha - see Self

qualification, s1, s5 - s13, s42
quantum physics, s23

raga, s21, s22
Raja Yoga, s9, p22, s92
rationality, s56
rejuvenation, s6
relationships, s10
relaxation, p24
religion, s65
representational systems, s21
resistance, s87
responsibility, s63
revelation, 20
    See also intuition
right action, s67
ritual, s65
R-complex, s5, s6, n1

sadhana, s12, p22, s65, s93, s96, s102

diet, and, s53
samadhi, p15, s65, s75, s89, s90
samahita yoga, p15, p22, s68, s102 - s108
sambhogakaya, s16
sakshatkara, p29
samskaras, s21
sat, s23
satya, s45
satyagraha, s10
science, s14, s26, s27, s49, s56
Self, s2, s11, s15, s16, s21, s23 - s25, s47, s68, s82
selflessness, s50
self-realization, s36
senses - modalities, and strategies, s21
sensory-motor mind, s21
separation, s51
service, selfless, s60
shakti, s3 - s5, s15, s16, s23
    Divine Mother, as, s79
shaktipat, s53, s69, s70, s71
    See also initiation
sharing, s57
sheaths, s14, s24, s25, s53
shiva, s15, s16, s23
shravana, p27
Schumann waves, s18, s19
siddhis, s67
six mental enemies, s12
six treasures, s6
sixth sense, s54
skilful action, s49, s56, s60, s80
specialness, s55, s57
speech, s13
spinal (*sumeru*) breath, p25
spirit, s23
spiritual crisis, p19
spiritual guide, s50, s52, s56
spiritual path, p17, s94, s102
spiritual preceptor, teacher; see guru
spirituality, s26, s27
strategic planning, s78, n9
stress, s17, s27
struggle, s83
subject - object consciousness, s61, s62, s63, s90
subjective experience, s28
submodalities, s21, s22, s47
subpersonalities, n7
subtle body, s18
superconsciousness, see *turiya*
surrender, s12, p23, s51, s98, s105
surya svara, s20

sutra format, p19, p29
svara yoga, s19, s20
sympathetic nervous system (SNS), s17, s20
synchronicity, s79, s80, s85, s87
summary of the path, s102 - s108

tantra, s6, s15, s16, s23
tapas, s12
teaching, the dangers of, s57
therapy, s21, s22
three shifts, the, s81, s85
tomato effect, s84
Tradition of the Himalayan Masters, p20
transpersonal visioning, s76 - s87, p139, n9, n10
Truth, see Centre of Consciousness
truthfulness, s10
turiya, s6, s25

ultradian rhythms, s19, s20
unconscious mind, s22, s67, s84
universe, in manifesting, s79, s85, s86
upliftment, s50, s52
urges, the four, s13, s17, s53

vairagya, p22, s65, s68
vanaprastha, s58, s101
vidya, s24
visioning, s48, s75, s78, s80 - s84, s87, p139
V-K dissociation, p24, s93, s97
Voice of the Silence, s55

watchful waiting, s64
wisdom, s96
Witness, s51, s97
worship, s65, s69, s70, s71, s74, s99

yamas, s9, s10, p26, figure 1
Yoga of the Centre of Consciousness, p15
Yoga, p17, s75, s92
    ascension, and, p17, p18
    Bhakti, p23, s65, s74, s92, s93
    discipline, of, s92
    Himalayan Tradition of, s4, p20, s61, s93, s95
    Jnana, p23, p27, s11, s15, s17, s54, s67, s92, s93
    Karma, p23, s76 - s87, s93
    life, of, s92, s93, s96
    Raja, s9, p22, s92
    science of spirituality, as, s14, p17, s26, s27, s49, s56
    skill in action, as, s49, s56, s60, s80
    therapeutic, p24, s27

yogic illness, s11, s53
yoga nidra, s25

About The Authors

Born in Ontario, the Jerrys have pursued parallel careers as health care professionals. Dr. Martin is a physician-scientist with 30 years of experience as a university professor in teaching, research, administration and clinical care in internal medicine, oncology and immunology. Dr. Marian is a clinical psychologist with a background in nursing who has had 30 years of experience in teaching, research, clinical and administrative aspects of health psychology as well as psychosocial oncology and palliative care. Both have published extensively and lectured internationally in their fields of expertise. The Jerrys have enjoyed an eight-year career in international development as consultants to the World Health Organization.

The Jerrys have been students of yoga since 1971. They began their studies with Vishnudevananda at the Sivananda Ashram in Montreal, and subsequently studied Transcendental Meditation, and then with the Self-Realization Fellowship (tradition of Paramahansa Yogananda). In 1982 they met their spiritual teacher, Swami Veda Bharati (premonastic name: Dr. Usharbudh Arya), who initiated them and their two sons into the Tradition of the Himalayan Masters. He introduced them in 1985 to their Spiritual Master, H.H. Sri Swami Rama of the Himalayas, who initiated them further. The Jerrys studied with their spiritual preceptors in India and at the Himalayan Institute in Honesdale, PA, USA, and in 1988 they hosted an international yoga congress for the Tradition in Calgary, Canada. At that time they established the Foothills Yoga Society in Calgary under the guidance of Swami Rama and Dr. Arya for which they have served as founding teachers.

Under the guidance of Swami Rama the Jerrys initiated the Himalayan Rural Health Development Project through the Division of International Development at the University of Calgary. This was a Canadian International Development Agency (CIDA) sponsored primary health development project in villages in the Himalayan foothills in partnership with the Himalayan Institute Hospital Trust founded by Swami Rama in Rishikesh, India. This experience has been the source of their interests in medical applications of yoga philosophy, psychology and practice and their clinical and laboratory research on the effects of meditation in cancer patients.

Printed in Great Britain
by Amazon.co.uk, Ltd.,
Marston Gate.